CHARITY CARE
TOOLS TO MANAGE THE UNINSURED POPULATION

Sandra J. Wolfskill, FHFMA

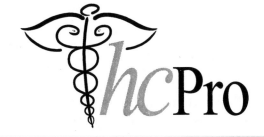

Sandra J. Wolfskill, FHFMA, Author
Deborah Datte, Esq., Contributor
Melissa Osborn, Senior Managing Editor
Jacqueline Diehl Singer, Layout Artist
Jean St. Pierre, Creative Director
Paul Singer, Layout Artist
Tom Philbrook, Cover Designer
Paul Nash, Group Publisher
Suzanne Perney, Publisher

Arrangements can be made for quantity discounts. For more information, contact:

HCPro, Inc.
P.O. Box 1168
Marblehead, MA 01945
Telephone: 800/650-6787 or 781/639-1872
Fax: 781/639-2982
E-mail: *customerservice@hcpro.com*

Visit HCPro at its World Wide Web sites:
www.hcpro.com and **www.hcmarketplace.com**

TABLE OF CONTENTS

CONTENTS

Chapter 5: Best practices: The ideal revenue cycle and charity processing . . .85

CONTENTS

ABOUT THE AUTHOR

Sandra J. Wolfskill, FHFMA

Sandra J. Wolfskill, FHFMA, is president of Wolfskill & Associates, Inc., a firm dedicated to quality healthcare receivables consulting. Prior to founding the firm in 1996, Sandra spent 15 years in healthcare financial management and consulting, including holding positions of vice president, senior consultant, director of patient financial services, director of information systems, and chief financial officer. Sandra has presented programs to national healthcare financial management conferences, as well as conducting seminars and training sessions throughout the United States.

Sandra's healthcare financial management and consulting activities have included the following:

- Conducting operational assessments for healthcare clients
- Facilitating the reengineering of the revenue cycle process for healthcare facilities in several states
- Preparing and presenting a variety of customized staff training programs for healthcare clients
- Developing and conducting customized, focused process re-evaluations for healthcare providers
- Serving as cofaculty for a National HFMA Receivables Management course
- Developing criteria-based position descriptions for patient financial service positions in compliance with JCAHO standards
- Organizing and managing all aspects of the financial operations of an acute care hospital
- Implementing receivables process redesign and imposed staffing reductions without adversely impacting levels of receivables or customer service
- Preparing policy and procedural manuals for admitting, registration, billing, collection, accounts payable, payroll, purchasing, information systems, and general ledger functional areas

Sandra received her Bachelor of Arts degree cum laude from Wittenberg University, Springfield, OH, and her Master of Arts Degree from the University of Delaware. She is an Advanced Member of the Northeast Ohio Chapter, HFMA, and a Fellow in HFMA, with a specialty in patient financial services, and a member of both the National Association of Healthcare Access Managers and the American Association of Healthcare Administrative Management.

About the Contributor

Deborah A. Datte, Esq.

Deborah A. Datte, Esq., is a partner with Post & Schell, PC, in Philadelphia. She is the former Vice President and General Counsel of Crozer Keystone Health System, has vast experience in sophisticated business transactions and taxation that have given her versatility, knowledge, and insight into the business of healthcare delivery. Her experience covers healthcare mergers and acquisitions, joint ventures between hospitals and their strategic partners, working and capital finance, and general corporate affairs. Drawing upon her Masters in Taxation, Datte also assists tax-exempt healthcare clients with excess benefit transaction determinations, issues associated with tax-exempt bonds, unrelated busines income, and other exempt organization concerns. She also possesses considerable experience forming and advising ERISA health and welfare benefit plans.

ACKNOWLEDGEMENTS

Compiling a book about healthcare charity practices never would have happened without the support and assistance of a wonderful group of healthcare clients, associates, and friends, including Alex McFadden, Larry Morris, Sandy Piersol, Cindy Ankrom, Wanda Diethelm, Ollivene Hickman, Rita Tracey, Marilyn Lipka, Gretchen Speicher, and Cheryl McMillan. The HCPro editors, especially Lori Levans, for promoting the book concept, and Melissa Osborn, for providing fantastic editorial assistance, made this project fun. Responsibility for any errors or omissions, is, of course, mine.

Sandra J. Wolfskill
Chardon, OH

1 ONE

Introduction to charity-care issues

Introduction to charity-care issues

The human equation

Healthcare billing and collection practices are complex. Until recently, the term "patient friendly" applied to clinicians and registration representatives, not to the patient billing process. The collections side of the process was all about collecting the most dollars possible and holding bad debts and charity deductions to the lowest possible levels. Few patient financial services directors and chief financial officers became involved in the human side of the equation, and patients with little or no health insurance were caught in a system they did not understand and in which they were unable to obtain the help they needed.

The New York Times, December 19, 2004,[1] reported one example of hospital collection practices that reflects badly on the healthcare industry. To paraphrase the story:

> Mrs. X left for work one day, leaving her sick husband at home. He had been hospitalized on several occasions and probably should have gone to the emergency department on that day, but he chose not to because the family owed more than $40,000 to the local hospital. The family had had no health insurance for years, and Mrs. X had only recently obtained insurance through her employer. She worked at a low-paying job, so she was not able to pay for family coverage.

Each time the family used the services of the local hospital, Mrs. X asked about any financial assistance that might help her family. She was consistently told that no assistance was available.

When she came home that evening, Mrs. X found that her husband had died.

Three months later, the hospital sued Mrs. X for the money her family owed. It obtained a judgment to garnish Mrs. X's wages. The hospital took $100 out of each paycheck; Mrs. X now only earned $680 (gross) every two weeks.

The family lost their trailer and moved to an apartment, and Mrs. X had to skip taking medications in order to keep it.

Mrs. X finally obtained legal help and convinced a judge to overturn the garnishment. The hospital was ordered to repay the money garnished, and eventually it did—after several months.

Meanwhile, an outside collection agency hired by the hospital pursued payment of other bills not included in the legal case.

Was this an isolated case or part of a common pattern of patient and hospital interaction? Until the lawsuits filed in 2004 against more than 400 hospitals and the American Hospital Association (AHA), public attention to the issues surrounding uncompensated care and hospital billing and collection practices was limited. However, as the number of uninsured individuals continues to rise, and as managed care plans are being redesigned to move more first-dollar responsibility (i.e., deductibles, or the amounts patients are required to pay before their healthcare insurance begins making payments) to patients, hospitals are facing increased pressure to revise their policies and procedures, especially their charity-care practices.

No one will argue that hospitals, even nonprofit hospitals, should operate at a loss. To do so long term could result in the collapse of the healthcare system. The balancing act involves hospitals' need to generate operating margins (profits) in order to expand and update capital and programs v. the need to care for those who cannot afford the services they require. Each hospital looks at charity care in light of its mission and value statements; the challenge is to operationally comply with the mission and, at the same time, support the financial viability of the organization.

Uncompensated care

Healthcare financial managers face the increasing challenge of managing not only revenue and expenses, but also uncompensated care. Uncompensated care represents services provided to patients for which the provider receives no payment. There are two classifications of uncompensated care:

- *Bad debt* accounts are defined as accounts where the responsible party has the ability to pay but does not do so in a timely manner or without intervention from an external collection agency.

- *Charity* accounts are accounts where the responsible party does not have the ability to pay based on a defined set of income and asset criteria. Providers may discount charity accounts fully or partially, based on income qualification guidelines.

Uncompensated care by the numbers

Hospitals have traditionally structured their charity programs to the Federal Poverty Guidelines (FPG), which the government updates annually. However, in the past few years, there has been a trend to expand the charity eligibility to greater percentages of the FPG (Figure 1.1).

Figure	1.1	Charity-care eligibility: Scale options

% of FPG	Single scale	Complex scale
100%	Base scale only	
150%	Base scale only	
200%		Sliding scale
400%		Sliding scale
600%		Sliding scale

With the ability to offer discounts to uninsured and underinsured patients, sliding scales are becoming a common tool for determining eligibility.

Uncompensated care as a percentage of expenditures has remained relatively constant, ranging from a high of 5.8% in 2000 to a low of 5.1% in 2002 (Figure 1.2).

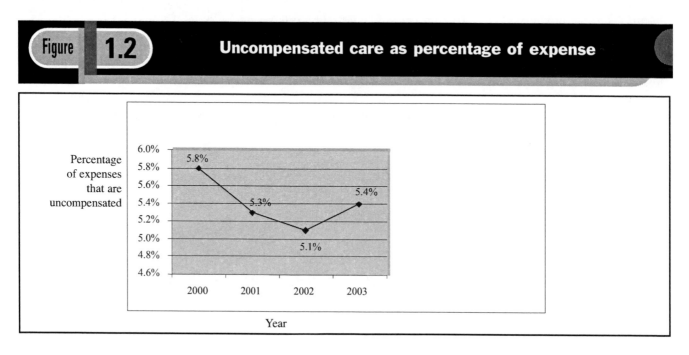

Figure 1.2 — **Uncompensated care as percentage of expense**

At the same time, the amount of uncompensated care provided has increased from a low of $21.5 billion dollars in 2001 to $24.9 billion dollars in 2003 (Figure 1.3).

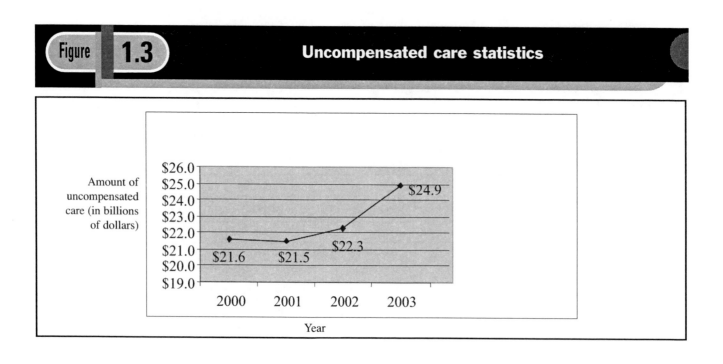

Figure 1.3 — **Uncompensated care statistics**

On an adjusted patient day basis, the cost to healthcare providers has followed a similar pattern, ranging from a low of $69.51 per adjusted patient day in 2001 to $78.75 per adjusted patient day in 2003 (Figure 1.4).

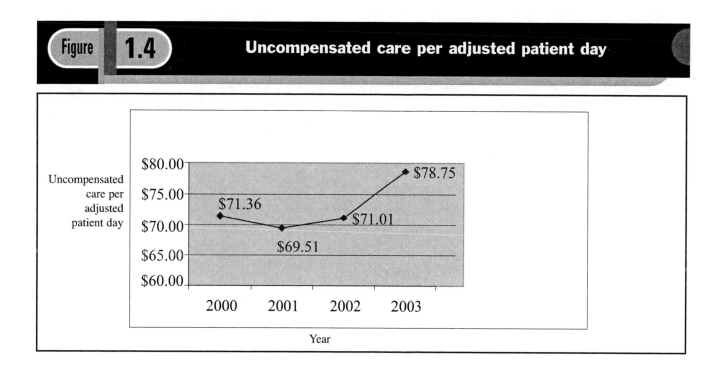

Figure 1.4 Uncompensated care per adjusted patient day

With hospital operating margins in 2003–2004 ranging from -1.84% to 4.1%, the incorporation of contemporary uncompensated care processing is an important aspect of healthcare financial management.

Reasons for increased uncompensated care

Why has uncompensated care become a major issue confronting American hospitals? One indicator that directly parallels the uncompensated care dollars is the number of individuals in poverty, which peaked in the early 1990s, declined, and increased again as the recession of 2000–2001 unfolded. According to the most recent Census data, in 2003, 35.9 million people lived in poverty, an increase of 1.3 million from 2002.

The second measure of poverty in the United States is the FPG, which the Department of Health and Human Services (HHS) publishes annually. The government and other organizations use these guidelines for administrative purposes, typically for determining eligibility for certain federal programs and provider charity discounts. Programs, including charity policies, may use percentage multiples of the guidelines (e.g., 200% of the guidelines) for determining full and partial eligibility. As Figure 1.5 illustrates, the FPG for a family of four has risen in each of the past five years.

At the same time as the increased FPG, the number of Americans without health insurance rose to an all-time high of 45 million people in 2003. This represents a 1.4 million increase in uninsured individuals in just one year.

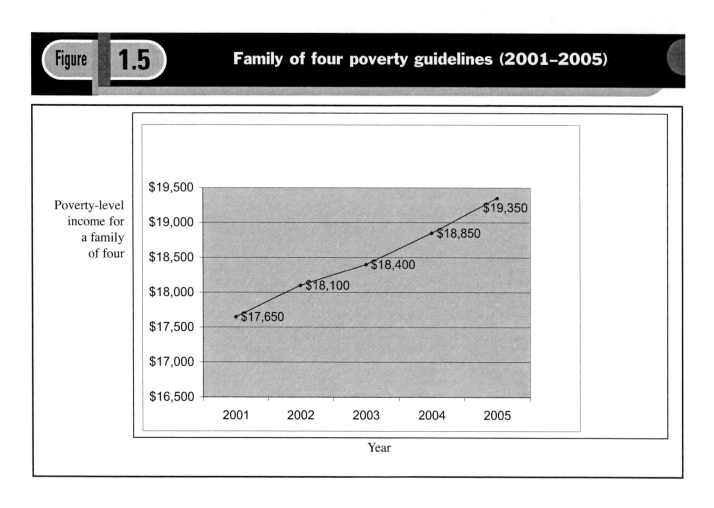

Figure 1.5 — Family of four poverty guidelines (2001–2005)

How hospital charges impact uninsured patients

What does this increase in the poverty guidelines and the number of uninsured Americans mean to patients without insurance?

The charge structures that hospitals developed during the "lesser of cost or charges" era, when government and commercial payer contracts penalized providers if their charges were less than the actual costs, has directly impacted uninsured individuals. Therefore, mark ups eventually exaggerated the true cost of any service or supply.

In an effort to control healthcare costs, government payers imposed prospective payment systems on providers, which further negated the value of charge structures as a true representation of cost. At the same time, commercial payers negotiated a variety of payment methodologies, all based on some form of discounting. In the end, hospitals only expected the patients without insurance to pay their full charges.

Changes in the charity-care arena

Until 2004, hospitals maintained that certain provisions of the Medicare program prohibited the use of discounts for self-pay patients. On December 16, 2003, Richard Davidson, president of the AHA, sent a letter to HHS Secretary Tommy Thompson in which the AHA maintained that Medicare program rules, as well as restrictions set out by the Office of Inspector General (OIG), made it virtually impossible for hospitals to offer discounts to low-income or medically indigent patients.

Secretary Thompson responded on February 19, 2004, refuting the AHA's charges and opening the door to major revisions in hospital charity policies and procedures. The Secretary directed the Centers for Medicare & Medicaid Services (CMS) and the OIG to provide guidance to hospitals on the topics of discounting and billing requirements for uninsured and underinsured patients:

> Your letter suggests that HHS regulations require hospitals to bill all patients using the same schedule of charges and suggests that as a result, the uninsured are forced to pay "full price" for their care. That suggestion is not correct and certainly does not accurately reflect my policy. The advice you have been given regarding this issue is not consistent with my understanding of Medicare's billing rules. To be sure that there will be no further confusion on this matter, at my direction, the Centers for Medicare & Medicaid Services and the Office of Inspector General have prepared summaries of our policy that hospitals can use to assist the uninsured and underinsured. This guidance shows that hospitals can provide discounts to uninsured and underinsured patients who cannot afford their hospital bills and to Medicare beneficiaries who cannot afford their Medicare cost-sharing obligations. Nothing in the Medicare program rules or regulations prohibit such discounts. In addition, the Office of Inspector General informs me that hospitals have the ability to offer discounts to uninsured and underinsured individuals and cost-sharing waivers to financially needy Medicare beneficiaries.[2]

Thus, the secretary and HHS went on record as allowing discounts to uninsured patients and underinsured patients. In addition, the waiver of cost-sharing payments from Medicare patients who were unable to pay and the determination of medical indigence paved the way for major revisions in hospital charity policies and practices. We present the discounting issue in greater detail in Chapter 2.

Charity-care policies and procedures

As a result of the position statements issued by HHS and the OIG, hospitals have updated their charity-care policies and procedures. A recent HCPro survey indicated that 65% of the respondents revised their charity processes within the past six months. In the same survey, 69% of the respondents indicated that the most recent revision of their charity policy has resulted in an increase in the charity dollars approved in their institutions.

Recently, a three-hospital system in Massachusetts announced a significant change in its charity policy and procedures. It plans to offer a discount of 35% to patients who do not qualify for public assistance but whose income falls between 401% and 600% of the FPG.

Comparing charity dollars to bad debt dollars as a percentage of net revenue confirms that bad debt write-offs continue to exceed charity write-offs by significant numbers. A recent HCPro survey provided the comparison in Figure 1.6:

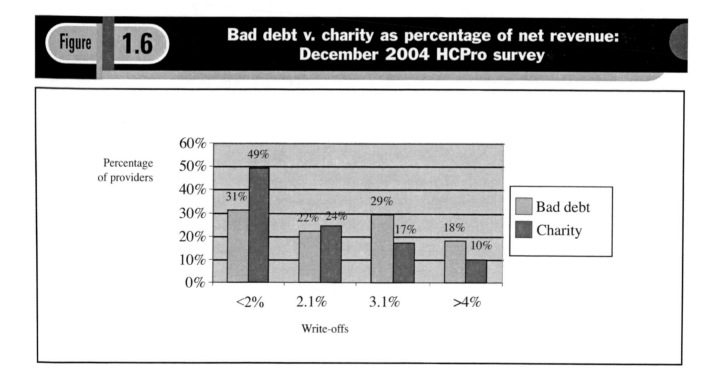

Figure 1.6

Bad debt v. charity as percentage of net revenue: December 2004 HCPro survey

In fact, 73% of the charity write-offs are valued at less than 3% of net revenue, whereas only 53% of the bad debt write-offs are in the same range. Charity and bad debt percentages appear to be inversely related; thus, charity write-offs tend to decrease as the value of bad debt placements increase. This data suggests that either more patients who can pay are not doing so—thus the bad debt placements—or hospitals are quicker to send accounts to collection than to approve charity write-offs.

Budget limitations do not appear to drive charity approval decisions. In the HCPro survey, 78% of the hospitals reported that write-offs are not limited by an approved budget amount. This lack of limitation is consistent with the definition of charity care, which speaks to the patient's inability to pay for the services provided.

Public education for charity services

Hospitals are increasingly using the media, including the Internet, to educate the public and provide information about their charity funding. According to one hospital Web site,

> In fiscal year 1998 alone, East Texas Medical Center (ETMC) provided $95 million in charity and uncompensated care. That's an average of $260,000 a day benefiting the people and communities of East Texas.

> Obviously, the need for care is great, and it is growing. It is up to all of us to answer that need. Across the nation, the cost of medical care continues to increase, while governmental health reform and managed care further decrease reimbursement for health services. In addition, East Texas' projected growth and aging population will continue to increase the demand for medical services and charitable care.

> It is our mission to serve all members of the community, regardless of race, creed, sex, national origin, handicap or ability to pay. That is why each year ETMC significantly exceeds the charity care requirement mandated for not-for-profit health organizations under state law.[3]

Another provider's Web site disclosed the following:

> As a nonprofit health care company, charity care is an important component of our service. In 2003, Banner provided $49.8 million in charity care to disadvantaged patients.[4]

However, other providers make no mention of charity care or free care on their Web sites. A few provider Web sites provided telephone numbers for patients to call and request financial assistance. The industry is all over the map when it comes to reporting charity care, publicly disclosing the availability of charity care, and clearly identifying how charity care impacts individual institutions.

Patient awareness of charity care

Patient awareness of the availability of charity care is also not universal. A recent study by the Center for Studying Health System Change (HSC) asked the uninsured about their awareness and use of healthcare providers offering lower cost and affordable care. Specifically, the study asked uninsured patients, "At this place, do you pay full price for medical care or do you pay a lower amount based on what you can afford to pay?" and "Thinking of the area where you live, is there a place that offers affordable medical care for people without insurance?"

The responses to these questions indicate that more than half of the uninsured (52%) are not aware of and do not use providers who provide such assistance in their communities. This also suggests that this significant portion of the population may be at increased risk of not pursuing needed medical services.

Survey participants did not identify hospitals as the primary safety net for the uninsured. In general, participants most often identified physicians, clinics, and health centers as sources of low-cost care. Specifically, 45% of the uninsured received healthcare from clinics or health centers, and 26% identified a physician office as their main source of healthcare. Only 8% of those surveyed identified the hospital emergency department (ED) as their primary healthcare safety net. However, other HSC research has shown that, in general, the uninsured receive more than half of their outpatient care from hospital-based facilities. In addition, typically 25% of all outpatient visits to hospitals by the uninsured are ED visits.

The HSC survey report concluded with the following observations:

> That more than half of the uninsured are unaware of safety net providers in the communities may also reflect the fact that so few identify hospital-based outpatient settings as sources of lower-cost care. While visits to hospital outpatient and emergency departments make up more than half of all outpatient visits by uninsured people, a comparatively smaller number of uninsured identified hospital-based facilities as safety net providers. Since services received in hospital-based settings are usually more expensive than in clinics or private physician offices, the uninsured may not perceive that hospitals are lower-cost sources of care, even if the services are provided at a discounted rate.[5]

Concerns have also been raised about some hospitals charging uninsured patients more than insured patients, implementing stringent eligibility standards for uncompensated care, and using aggressive bill collection practices as a way to discourage future use, all of which may add to the perception among many uninsured people that hospitals are not sources of lower-cost medical care.[6]

How EMTALA affects charity-care policies

All Medicare-participating hospitals that offer emergency services must comply with the Emergency Medical Treatment and Labor Act (EMTALA). Passed by Congress in 1986, this act ensures access to emergency services regardless of an individual's ability to pay. Hospitals with EDs must provide a medical screening examination whenever a patient arrives in the ED and requests the examination or is in labor, regardless of the individual's ability to pay. Thereafter, hospitals are required to provide stabilizing treatment or appropriate transfer if the patient requests the transfer or if the hospital is unable to stabilize the patient within its capability.

How do the EMTALA rules affect hospital charity-care practices? Patient access staff must be careful that there is no suggestion of a link between the patient's ability to pay and the hospital's provision of services. To this end, many providers have implemented abbreviated initial registration activities, followed by a comprehensive patient discharge process upon completion of the ED services.

The 2003 EMTALA regulations permit hospitals to follow a reasonable registration process, including asking for demographic, insurance, and emergency contact information, as long as that inquiry does not delay screening or treatment. However, there is also the caveat that the registration process may not unduly discourage patients from remaining for additional evaluation and treatment.

Tax-exempt status—Federal level

A significant issue for many nonprofit hospitals is their federal, state, and local tax-exempt status. For federal purposes, status as a 501(c)(3) organization requires that the organization meet specific regulatory and statutory requirements. Beginning with the articles of incorporation and bylaws, the organization must establish its existence as an exclusively charitable organization. The organization should prohibit substantial unrelated business activity not associated with the organization's exempt purposes.

The organization may participate in a limited number of unrelated business activities, as long as those activities are an insignificant part of the organization's total activities. The government then taxes revenue from the unrelated activities as unrelated business income.

To qualify for tax-exempt status, the organization must provide a public service or serve the public interest. The organization must also prove that it does not benefit private individuals. In order words, profits may not accrue to private individuals, only to the corporation as a whole.

Criteria for tax-exempt status

The community benefit standard (Revenue Rule 69-545) looks at the following factors in relation to a hospital's tax-exempt status:

- Does the hospital offer emergency services to all individuals without regard to their ability to pay for those services? *Note:* The EMTALA regulations require this of all hospitals with dedicated EDs.

- Does a community board govern the hospital?

- Does the hospital maintain an open medical staff?

- Does the hospital provide nondiscriminatory treatment for Medicare and Medicaid patients?

- Does the hospital serve a broad spectrum of the community such that the community obtains a benefit from the hospital's existence? If the organization uses charity care write-offs to meet the community benefit standard, it must document the amount of charity care provided.

There has been a presumption by the Internal Revenue Service (IRS) that collection efforts may undercut the status of charity care for nonprofit hospitals. However, in the St. David's Health Care System case, the federal court held that "charitable services may include collection attempts as long as patients who were found unable to pay their bills often had them reduced or entirely canceled."[7]

For the majority of nonprofit hospitals, the issue is not *meeting* these requirements, but rather providing the public and government agencies with sufficient information to *demonstrate* meaningful compliance. The IRS form 990 reporting requirement is important because, under IRS regulations, tax-exempt organizations are required to make available the community benefit information to anyone requesting that information.

Disclosure of charity-care dollars

Nonprofit hospitals derive their tax-exempt status in part from the provision of charity care. But how much charity care do hospitals provide? That is a fundamental question driving the discussion on this issue. Hospitals typically track the amount of charity care provided, but disclosing the basis for the total dollars reported and publicly reporting total dollars are different issues.

According to a Modern Healthcare survey in June 2004, most hospitals do not report charity care in their public disclosures, even though the IRS requires "complete" disclosure of charity provided. Even when the hospital reports the dollars of charity care, there are no standard reporting criteria to enable the reader to know whether the figures provided are gross charges or the actual cost of the charity care provided. According to the HCPro survey, only 78% of the respondents indicated that their facilities report charity dollars on the annual IRS 990 forms.

The issue of a lack of standardized reporting is highlighted by the following data from the HCPro survey:

What is included in your facility's definition of charity for tax reporting purposes?

Volunteer hours	13%
Health screenings	39%
Community service hours	35%
Charity deductions from revenue	94%
Other	10%

Congressional hearings for charity care

In 2004, several congressional committees began investigating hospital billing and collection practices, as well as hospital charging practices and the tax-exemption issue. First, on June 22, 2004, the House Committee on Ways and Means Subcommittee on Oversight held hearings on the tax-exemption issue. Although there are more than 300,000 tax-exempt 501(c)(3) entities, hospitals represent only 1.9% of this total number of entities. However, hospitals account for 41% of the total expenditures. Industry estimates place 80–85% of all hospitals into the tax-exempt category. Citing this data, the committee chairman opened hearings on two topics: healthcare charity practices and hospital pricing practices.

A key question posed by the committee chairman related to the ability to differentiate between for-profit and nonprofit hospitals. Testimony from several experts agreed that the market practices of the nonprofit hospitals are different from that of the for-profit institutions. There was also consensus that the determining factors of a hospital's qualification as nonprofit should go beyond the issue of charity care or uncompensated care to include the institution's role in the community, community service, etc. Finally, the panel agreed to make more information available to the public involving cost and quality.

Healthcare industry representatives provided testimony concerning costs and pricing strategies, noting that charges are often a byproduct of negotiated discount and fee arrangements. Also, charges only distantly relate to cost. Thus, nonprofit providers have developed mechanisms to deal with uninsured and underinsured patients. Aggressive discounting to this group of patients was cited during the hearings as one solution to the cost/charge dilemma.

The initial hearing was basically a fact-finding effort, which also highlighted the fact that individual nonprofit hospitals have vastly different charity-care practices.

Two days later, on June 24, 2004, the House Committee on Energy and Commerce Subcommittee on Oversight and Investigations opened hearings to follow up on letters sent in July 2003 to 20 of the largest hospital systems. In the fact-finding request letter, the committee indicated that they are

> ". . . conducting an investigation into the billing practices of certain medical providers under which the uninsured are expected to pay substantially higher amounts for medical services than third party health plans such as medical insurers, health maintenance organizations and preferred provider organizations (collectively, "third party health plans"), or government health care programs. These practices raise significant public health and consumer protection issues. The uninsured seem caught in the middle of the sophisticated and complicated forces driving health care financing including government entitlements, managed care, rising costs and shrinking public funds."[8]

The letter went on to discuss the uniform chargemaster requirement, the inflation of charges above costs, and the lack of discounting to uninsured patients. The 20 items requested by the committee represent a substantial data collection effort. The committee had not published the complete transcript and data analysis as of January 2005.

The stated purpose of the committee was to reduce the rates charged to uninsured patients. The committee recommended tying rates charged to the uninsured to the discounted rates given to managed care payers. Testimony from Herb Kuhn, director for CMS' Center for Medicare Management, repeated CMS' position that Medicare program rules and billing requirements do not prohibit discounts as long as the provider reports full charges on the cost report and maintains records, as in any business. Further, indigency rules do not prevent discounting to uninsured, and providers can make medical indigency determinations. Finally, he reconfirmed that the Medicare rules do not require providers to be aggressive in the collection of accounts. However, the regulations do require similar treatment of Medicare and non-Medicare accounts.

Other testimony suggested that Congress could require hospitals to provide patients with information about payment options when admitted, which should benefit the uninsured. Mark Rukavina, executive director of the Access Project, a group that supports organizations seeking to improve access to healthcare, stated his group's frustration at the lack of written information available from providers to patients about payment options, collection processes, and discounts.

Summary

The number of uninsured individuals as well as the steady increase in the federal poverty levels evidences the need for charity care. Nonprofit hospitals have a huge incentive to provide charity care as part of their efforts to meet the community benefit standard for maintaining their tax-exempt status. The 2004 CMS clarifications concerning discounting to uninsured and underinsured patients has opened the door for significant revisions to charity and discounting practices; the challenge for providers is to implement meaningful change while also protecting the financial viability of their organizations.

Notes

1. The names of the family members, communities, and hospital have been eliminated.

2. Text of letter from Tommy G. Thompson, secretary of HHS, to Richard J. Davidson, president, AHA. This can be found at *www.dhhs.gov/news/press/2004pres/20040219.html*.

3. *www.etmc.org/page.php?pageID=465*.

4. *www.bannerhealth.com/media/finance+information.asp*.

5. Issue Brief No. 90, November 2004, Center for Studying Health System Change.

6. See Note 4.

7. 349 F.3d 232, 236n3 (5th Cir. 2003)

8. *http://energycommerce.house.gov/108/News/07162003_1040.htm*.

Legal background

Legal background

Written by Deborah Datte, Esq.
Partner
Post & Schell, P.C.
Philadelphia

Although programs such as Medicaid and the State Children's Health Insurance Program provide healthcare coverage to the poorest Americans, it is estimated that more than 45 million Americans remain uninsured. These numbers signal a national healthcare crisis. Many of the uninsured are individuals who do not have access to affordable insurance through their employer and will not otherwise qualify for government entitlement programs, but there is also a large segment of the population, often self-employed individuals, who voluntarily choose to forego insurance coverage.

Who is responsible for the uninsured? Public sentiment seems to be increasingly turning to the nonprofit healthcare sector, whose tax exemptions basically provide a public subsidy. The recent developments described in this chapter are forcing healthcare organizations to rethink the way they bill the uninsured and administer their charity-care programs.

Hospital charges

As a preliminary matter, it must be noted that hospital charges are an accounting convention exclusive to the hospital industry. Because many payers, including Medicare and managed care organizations, base hospital reimbursement on case rates or diagnosis-related groups, a hospital's charges become less important. However, when payers reimburse hospitals based on a percentage of the hospital's charges, the hospital's chargemaster becomes far more significant.

Hospital charges are a concern with respect to several Medicare reimbursement issues, including outlier payments (both inpatient and outpatient), new technology, brachytherapy seeds, and those remaining cost-reimbursed areas where the apportionment formula still applies. The Centers for Medicare & Medicaid Services (CMS) has indicated that charge discounting to the uninsured or underinsured, done within the scope of the February and June 2004 guidance letters, will not cause compliance or payment problems. Why? CMS has indicated that in the case of outliers, the cost-to-charge ratio used is always from the most recently filed cost report. Providers must report full, uniform charges on the Medicare cost report. This reporting of full charges on the cost report is the core practice that all hospitals must maintain.

The uniformity of charges requirement is important to CMS because it commutes its statistics, such as the cost-to-charge ratio, based on full charges. Further, PRM 2203 clearly indicates that providers may charge whatever they want as long as they comply with the uniform charge requirement for cost reporting to Medicare. Translated, this means that if a hospital discounts reference laboratory charges, those charges must be adjusted back to the uniform gross amounts when reported on the cost report. However, as discussed later in this chapter, the CMS and Office of Inspector General (OIG) guidance on discounting to the uninsured and underinsured indicates that such discounting of charges is acceptable, within the limitations indicated in the guidance documents. This subject will be further discussed later in this chapter.

Class-action litigation and the uninsured

Hospital charity-care practices came to the forefront in mid-2004, when more than 40 not-for-profit (and several for-profit) hospitals and health systems were named as defendants in a national class-action lawsuit. Richard Scruggs, founder of The Scruggs Law Firm in Mississippi, was the architect of the charity-care class-action lawsuits. He also masterminded the beginnings of the tobacco litigation that in 1998 resulted in one of the largest class-action settlements in American history.[1] Scruggs and law firms working with The Scruggs Law Firm filed the first suits in June 2004 against 13 hospitals/health systems in seven states. Since then, counsel has filed more than 40 suits in federal court in 22 states. Additional cases making almost identical state law claims have been filed in state courts throughout the country.

Scruggs' charity-care class-action suits generally allege that the defendant hospitals and health systems failed to provide adequate levels of uncompensated care, targeted the uninsured with improper collection efforts, and charged the uninsured significantly more for their care than the insured were charged.

The massive litigation effort is well organized. The Scruggs Law Firm and the firms with which it works maintain a Web site[2] that, among other things, actively recruits uninsured individuals to act as the named plaintiff and class representative in future class action suits using an online questionnaire. The firm systematically issues press releases with each new round of complaints, ensuring that the litigation is placed before an ever-growing pool of potential representative plaintiffs. The Web site also contains a PowerPoint presentation entitled "Litigation Against Profiteering Nonprofit Hospitals," which speaks to the evils perpetrated by hospitals nationwide against the uninsured. The site also maintains copies of the complaints filed throughout the country, which plaintiffs' counsel can use as templates for future lawsuits.

Developments in the cases

While these cases were still in their infancy, North Mississippi Medical System (NMMS) entered into a preemptive settlement agreement with the Scruggs firm before the firm listed the system as one of the defendants in the barrage of class-action suits then pending. In the Memorandum of Understanding, NMMS agreed to do the following:

- Limit the amount it attempts to collect annually from an individual to 10% of that individual's annual income

- Provide free care to uninsured patients with incomes at or below 200% of the federal poverty level (FPL)

- Provide care to uninsured patients at the applicable Medicare rates or 51% of charges for services not covered by Medicare, and further discount those amounts for patients with incomes at or below 400% of the FPL

- Recalculate the bills of the uninsured for services provided within three years and 45 days of August 5, 2004, pursuant to the new charity-care guidelines, and refund any excess collected

- Pay plaintiffs' counsel's legal fees

Interestingly, NMMS also agreed to comply with provisions of the Sarbanes-Oxley Act, which are not generally applicable to nonprofit entities.

In September 2004, the Judicial Panel on Multi-District Litigation held a hearing to consider plaintiff counsel's requests to consolidate the cases filed in federal court throughout the country before a single court. This would allow the plaintiffs to pool their efforts into what amounts to a single action and, as was the case in the tobacco litigation, creates a sizable settlement pool.

In October 2004, the charity-care class action effort was dealt its first blow when the Judicial Panel on Multidistrict Litigation denied the plaintiffs' request for consolidation. Since the judicial panel's ruling, in response to motions to dismiss filed by the hospital and health systems defendants in federal cases throughout the country, one case after another has been dismissed, leaving plaintiffs with a decision to either re-file in state court with the limited state law claims that were originally asserted in federal actions or forego additional litigation altogether. Although it is likely that this trend will continue based on the weaknesses of the federal claims asserted, the state law claims made by plaintiffs are largely untried.

What are the allegations?

Each lawsuit names at least one uninsured individual who received services at the defendant hospital or health system as a plaintiff. The named plaintiff or plaintiffs represent an unnamed "class" of plaintiffs composed of the uninsured who received services from, and were billed by, the hospital defendant. Although the allegations against each of the plaintiff hospitals and health systems differ slightly based on the idiosyncrasies of state laws, the allegations typically fall into the following categories:

Breach of contract

The federal complaints employ a novel and untried theory that federal tax exemption creates a contract between an organization recognized as tax exempt pursuant to Section 501(c)(3) of the Internal Revenue Code and the federal government, as well as a contract between the hospital and the state and local governments that grant income, real estate, and sales tax exemptions. Federal, state, and local tax exemptions provide a public subsidy to exempt organizations, and those organizations are required to satisfy specific tests to maintain their exemption. State requirements differ from jurisdiction to jurisdiction.

Generally speaking, the complaints allege that the defendant hospitals and health systems breached their obligations as exempt organizations to do the following:

- Operate exclusively for charitable purposes

- Provide emergency room (ER) medical care without regard to the patient's ability to pay

- Provide affordable medical care to the uninsured

- Not pursue outstanding medical debt from the uninsured through aggressive collection practices

- Not allow charitable assets to impermissibly benefit private individuals and entities

The lawsuits employ a breach of contract theory in an attempt to create a private right of action against the hospitals under the Internal Revenue Code and state and local laws where none previously existed. The suits claim that the uninsured are third-party beneficiaries to the contracts between the hospitals and the federal, state, and local governments in which they operate. The suits also state that when an exempt hospital fails to fulfill its obligations under state and federal law, it is breaching its contracts with the government to the detriment of the individuals who should have benefited from the hospital's fulfillment of those obligations.

The complaints uniformly contain allegations that the defendant hospitals have breached their charity-care obligations and unfairly charged the uninsured by billing "sticker prices" that reflect grossly inflated charges rather than the deep discounts the hospitals offer insured patients. Some of the complaints allege that the defendant hospitals have distorted the amount of charity care they provide using "Enron-style accounting tricks." The complaints allege that hospitals aggressively use "abusive, harassing, and humiliating" collection practices against the uninsured. Inexplicably, many of the suits allege a further violation of these supposed contracts in that hospitals improperly allow non-charitable, for-profit physicians and vendors to use their facilities for profit-making purposes. The suits make these allegations notwithstanding the Internal Revenue Services' (IRS) long-standing requirement that tax-exempt hospitals maintain an open medical staff. Several of the complaints cite transfers of significant funds from the tax-exempt hospitals to taxable affiliates, and many allege that hospitals are extending preferential pricing to members of the hospitals' board of directors and other insiders.

Some of the complaints contain a second state law breach of contract claim based on form agreements that the uninsured are purportedly required to enter into with the hospital at the time that they receive care whereby the patient agrees to pay for care. These counts allege that there is an express or implied contractual obligation that the hospitals charge a fair and reasonable amount for the care provided and that the hospital breached this obligation when it billed patients full and "inflated" charges.

Breach of duty of good faith/fair dealing

Based on the implied or express contracts described above, the complaints allege that some or all of the following activities amount to bad faith and unfair dealing:

- Failing to provide ER care without regard to ability to pay

- Charging undiscounted and unreasonable charges, and charging the uninsured more than insured patients

- Using improper collection practices

- Allowing private physicians and other private parties to use exempt facilities

- Providing discounts to board members and other insiders

The most significant of these allegations is the second—that hospitals charge the uninsured significantly more than the insured. As a preliminary matter, it must be noted that hospital charges are an accounting convention exclusive to the hospital industry. Because many payers, including Medicare and managed care organizations, base hospital reimbursement on case rates or diagnosis-related groups, a hospital's charges become less important. However, when payers reimburse hospitals based on a percentage of the hospital's charges, the hospital's chargemaster becomes far more significant. For example, if a payer reimburses the hospital for outpatient services as 60% of charges, the higher the hospital's charges, the more the hospital will receive in payment. How meaningful charges are depends on the hospital's market (i.e., whether payers in the market base their payments on the hospital's charges). If payers reimburse the hospital based upon a case rate or another mechanism unrelated to hospital charges, those charges become irrelevant to hospital reimbursement.

Breach of charitable trust

The complaints allege that acceptance of federal, state, and local tax exemptions create a public charitable trust under federal and state law. Based on the factual allegations in the previous paragraph, the complaints allege that the defendant hospitals and health systems breached this charitable trust.

Violations of the Emergency Medical Treatment and Labor Act

Several of the complaints allege violations of the Emergency Medical Treatment and Labor Act (EMTALA), a law that, unlike the laws described above, explicitly provides for a private right of action. The complaints that include EMTALA counts claim that hospitals are conditioning medical screening examinations and treatment for emergency medical conditions on the plaintiffs' ability to pay and the provision of financial guarantees.

Constitutional and discrimination counts

A recent complaint filed against a Pennsylvania health system added a count alleging violations of Section 1983 and the 14th and 15th amendments of the U.S. Constitution to the previously used arsenal. These federal claims allege that the health systems acted under the auspices of federal and state law (e.g., the system's Medicare and Medicaid participation agreements, its reliance on Medicare and Medicaid disproportionate share payments and other charity-care subsidies, and the system's claim that it is legally required to collect charges from the uninsured) to deprive the uninsured of federally protected and constitutional rights.

Miscellaneous counts

Most of the complaints contain counts that claim unjust enrichment based on the argument that the hospitals obtained payments from the uninsured that exceeded what those hospitals should have charged. Many of the suits name the American Hospital Association (AHA) as a conspirator, and those complaints contain civil conspiracy and aiding and abetting counts. The counts against the AHA reference the recent correspondence between the AHA and Tommy Thompson, secretary of the Department of Health and Human Services, to support the proposition that the AHA assisted its tax exempt membership in falsely justifying the hospital's billing practices involving the uninsured. Most of the complaints allege that allowing the practices described above to continue will result in irreparable harm to the uninsured and the suits request injunctive relief (i.e., a court order precluding the defendant hospitals/health systems from charging the uninsured full charges and using aggressive collection practices against the uninsured). Many suits claim violations of state consumer protection and state and federal fair debt collection laws.

In addition to the injunctive relief that most of the suits request, the complaints request that the plaintiff class receive all damages suffered as a result of the conduct of the hospitals/health systems and that a constructive trust be imposed on the named hospitals' and health systems' tax savings, profits derived from charging the uninsured full charges, and assets and revenues sufficient to provide affordable care to the uninsured. Although attorney fees are not routinely requested in the complaints, federal law permits the court to award legal fees to plaintiffs' counsel.

Litigation that preceded the charity-care class-action lawsuits

In late 2002, a consumer advocacy group brought suit in California against the for-profit Tenet Healthcare Corporation, claiming that the system inappropriately billed Latino patients full charges while offering discounts to private and government insurers. The case settled for an undisclosed amount and Tenet agreed to implement a discount policy pending regulatory approval. The Tenet case resulted in a groundswell of press associated with the collection practices of hospitals against the uninsured.

In early 2003, the Connecticut attorney general filed suit against Yale–New Haven Hospital, claiming that the hospital misused "free bed" funds donated by the public. The suit sought a court order requiring the hospital to provide real and meaningful access to free bed funds for individuals who are unable to pay for their care, notice of the availability of the funds, elimination of barriers to apply for the funds, and elimination of debt collection efforts against those who qualify for free care. In response to the lawsuit, Yale–New Haven revised its charity-care policy to provide for discounts to the uninsured who earn between 250% and 350% of the federal poverty guidelines.

The government reaction to the uninsured

A solution to the health insurance crisis has been on the agenda of both the Clinton and the Bush administrations. President Clinton's first campaign focused on a national healthcare program, but his proposals died in Congress when they were characterized as socialized medicine. The Bush administration has chosen to take small steps, introducing pre-tax health savings accounts and tax incentives for employers to offer health insurance coverage to employees. It is impossible to know what impact these initiatives might have over time. Critics believe that employers will use health savings accounts as an excuse to eliminate employer-sponsored health insurance programs.

The immediate impact of the federal initiatives is negligible. A recent report published in *Health Affairs, the Policy Journal of the Health Sphere*,[3] estimated that one-half of federal bankruptcies filed were precipitated, at least in part, by medical debt. The report also estimates a significant increase in so-called "medical bankruptcy" in the 24 years preceding its publication. It is likely that as the ranks of the uninsured grow and voters demand resolution, the government's focus on the issue will intensify.

The Internal Revenue Service

Neither Section 501(c)(3) of the Internal Revenue Code nor the regulations interpreting it requires a tax-exempt hospital to provide charity care in order to obtain or maintain tax-exempt status. Rather, the concept of free or discounted care for those unable to pay for it first surfaced in a 1956 revenue ruling that required an unspecified level of charity care (i.e., free or discounted care) to be provided by hospitals as a condition to a grant and continuation of tax exemption.[4] By 1969, the IRS reversed its prior position on the basis that it was subjective and difficult to administer. Revenue Ruling 69-545 established a community benefit standard, the standard that continues to apply today.[5]

The IRS' community benefit standard requires that a tax-exempt hospital operate a full-time ER open to all persons, without regard to ability to pay. The standard also requires hospitals to have a board of directors drawn from the community, maintain an open medical staff, and apply any surplus to improving facilities, equipment, patient care, medical training, education, and research. The ruling explicitly recognized as exempt from federal taxation a hospital that (a) limited the class of individuals it would serve in non-emergency situations to persons able to pay the cost of that care, either by themselves, or through third-party reimbursement, and (b) referred non-emergency patients who could not meet its financial requirements for admission to other institutions that treated indigents.

Revenue Ruling 69-545 became the target of an unsuccessful class action challenge shortly after the IRS published it. On appeal, the District of Columbia Circuit upheld the more relaxed obligations for tax exemption described in the 1969 ruling and found that the community benefit standard did not eliminate the financial ability standard but rather provided an alternative to that standard.[6]

By the mid-1980s, charity care became an issue in connection with the grant of state tax exemptions, most notably in Utah, Pennsylvania, and Vermont. State legislation and common law in many jurisdictions requires the provision of specific levels of charity care by organizations that wish to benefit from exemption from state and local taxes. For example, Pennsylvania's Institutions of Purely Public Charity Act requires that one of several alternative financial assistance tests be satisfied as a condition to obtaining exemption from property and sales and use taxes.

In 1991, proposed federal legislation would have required exempt hospitals to annually provide charity care equivalent to 50% of the value of their tax exemption. Another bill would have required the provision of charity care equivalent to 5% of an exempt hospital's gross revenues as one of several alternative tests that would have to be satisfied to qualify for exemption. At hearings associated with these bills, representatives of the IRS testified that the community benefit standard espoused in Revenue Ruling 69-545 was a more appropriate measure of charitable status than the proposed financial requirements. Congress did not pass either bill.

Notwithstanding Revenue Ruling 69-545, courts have examined a hospital's charity-care activities as one (but not necessarily the dispositive) indicia of charitable status. Where charity care is an issue, courts have found that simply establishing a charity-care program, without more, is insufficient. The organization must actually provide charity care.[7] Using these court cases as a base, the IRS issued a non-binding field service advice to exempt organizations' branch auditors in February 2001 that concluded that the mere presence of charity-care policies was insufficient to satisfy the charity-care requirement of the community benefit standard, unless the hospital can demonstrate in practice that such policies actually "result in the delivery of significant healthcare services to the indigent."[8] Again, this advice is not binding on either the service or exempt organizations. It does, however, provide valuable insight into how the IRS may interpret its regulations.

In October 2004, the IRS published a new Application for Recognition of Exemption from Federal Income Taxation (Form 1023). Schedule C, the new application, applies to hospitals (including clinics and other organizations that provide medical care) and medical research organizations. Question five of the new Schedule C asks for much more detailed information respecting the organization's charity-care practices than the previous application.

State regulations

Many states directly and indirectly regulate the provision of uncompensated care. For example, Illinois' Community Benefits Act requires detailed reporting to the attorney general of uncompensated care and other community benefits. In Pennsylvania, virtually all eligible nonprofit hospitals participate in the Hospital Uncompensated Care program under the Tobacco Settlement Act of 2001. These laws, in turn, shape the policies and practices of tax-exempt hospitals.

Pennsylvania law clearly defines "uncompensated care" and related terminology, and it mandates basic hospital practices such as assisting eligible individuals to enroll in Medicaid. Importantly, Pennsylvania law requires hospitals to actively pursue the collection of claims for all possible sources of payment. Pennsylvania's highly structured program, differentiating between those patients who are unable to pay and those unwilling to pay, requires participating hospitals to develop clear institutional policies and practices. The treatment of uninsured patients in Pennsylvania may, therefore, differ from that of indigent patients in other states.

The federal response: CMS and the OIG

In response to public allegations that hospitals were inappropriately billing the uninsured and, in very rare cases, using collection practices that resulted in patients losing their homes or filing for protection under applicable bankruptcy laws, the AHA sent a letter to Tommy Thompson in late 2003 requesting relief from the regulatory climate that required hospitals to attempt to recover their charges from the uninsured. The letter stated, in part, that

> Hospitals believe that patients of limited means should not have to pay full charges simply because they have no coverage. But federal Medicare regulations as written today contain a string of barriers that discourage hospitals from reducing charges or forgiving debt for these patients without potentially running afoul of the law. And our members tell us that past experience with federal regulatory enforcement makes them extremely reluctant to risk it.[9]

Plaintiffs' counsel in the above-described class action lawsuits seized upon this letter, as well as several member publications issued by the AHA, in crafting the conspiracy counts in the class-action lawsuits that include the AHA as a named defendant. The plaintiffs argue that the AHA advised its members that they are legally required to bill the uninsured full charges and engage in aggressive collection activities, and therefore conspired with its member hospitals to act in the manner alleged in the complaints.

Thompson responded to the AHA's letter in February 2003. In his response, Thompson stated that the suggestion that federal regulations require hospitals to bill all patients using the same charge schedule and to force the uninsured to pay full charges is not correct and "certainly does not accurately reflect my policy." He attached policy guidance that he requested from CMS and the OIG in response to the AHA's letter. The guidance addressed the impact of the federal anti-kickback statute and the OIG's permissive exclusion authority on the offering of discounts to the uninsured and underinsured. That guidance generally provides the following:

- In the case of the anti-kickback statute, the law prohibits incentives for referrals of federal healthcare business, but it does not prohibit discounts to the uninsured who are otherwise unable to pay their hospital bills.

- In the case of discounts offered to the underinsured, the anti-kickback statute could be implicated if discounts are "tied directly or indirectly to the furnishing of items or services payable by a federal healthcare program."

- In the case of the government's permissive exclusion authority, the OIG may exclude a provider from participating in federal healthcare programs if that provider submits a request for payment to Medicare or Medicaid for amounts that are substantially more than the provider's usual charges.[10] This provision has been largely responsible for hospitals levying full charges on the uninsured. To the extent that a hospital routinely offers discounts from charges to the uninsured, its "usual charges" will likely be eroded.[11]

The guidance further states that the OIG has never exercised its exclusion authority against a provider who offered discounts to the uninsured or underinsured. To provide more comfort to the provider community in this regard, in September 2004 the OIG issued proposed regulations that would eliminate discounts for services provided to the uninsured and underinsured "free of charge or at a *substantially reduced rate*" from the calculation of usual charges.[12]

The guidance further stresses that until final regulations are released, the OIG will maintain an enforcement policy consistent with the proposed regulations. The guidance also addressed the safe harbor applicable to waiver of Medicare financial responsibility amounts in the case of beneficiaries who are unable to pay.[13]

However, what the OIG guidance does not address is the application of the usual and customary charges rule by payers other than federal healthcare programs. Many private payers have adopted rules similar if not identical to Medicare. Absent a modification of those rules or the provider agreement, in situations where a hospital is being paid for any services based upon a percentage of charges, a private payer could argue that the charges on which its payments are based should be reduced to reflect the discounts enjoyed under the hospital's charity-care policy.

The guidance skirted a discussion of Medicare's bad debt rules by stating that the OIG has not issued any regulations requiring hospitals to engage in any type of collection practices because enforcement of the bad debt rules falls within the purview of CMS.[14] Arguably, however, Medicare's bad debt rules would require a hospital to initiate the level of collection efforts against the uninsured as are required to be applied against Medicare beneficiaries under the bad debt rules. (See Testimony of Herb Kuhn discussed below.) These rules do not, however, speak to how much hospitals must charge patients.

The Congressional response

In 2003, subcommittees of both the House Ways and Means and the Energy and Commerce Committees commenced hearings regarding whether the government should impose more specific charity-care requirements on exempt organizations to justify the federal subsidies that their tax exemptions represent. Among the issues addressed at those hearings is the legal climate that has resulted in the hospital industry's practice of billing the uninsured based on full charges. Most notable among the individuals testifying before these subcommittees, for purposes of this discussion, were David Bernd, chairman of the AHA; Lewis Morris, chief counsel to the OIG; and Herb Kuhn, director for CMS' Center for Medicare Management.

In his testimony, Bernd described the AHA's principles and guidelines associated with hospital billing and collection practices. He addressed some of the issues raised in the complaints associated with disproportionate share and indirect medical education payments, noting that only a portion of America's hospitals enjoys these additional payments under the Medicare program and neither of these payments takes into account uncompensated care provided by those hospitals. He then spoke to the current requirements for hospital tax exemption, supporting the standards espoused in Revenue Ruling 69-545.

Morris' testimony reiterated the positions taken by the OIG in the guidance described above regarding application of the federal anti-kickback statute and the OIG's permissive exclusion authority. Kuhn testified that the methods by which a provider determines indigence with respect to non-Medicare patients should be similar to indigence determinations for Medicare beneficiaries. He also stated that in the case of bad debt, the collection efforts aimed at Medicare beneficiaries as a condition to including uncollected amounts on a provider's cost report should be on par with the collection efforts used for non-Medicare patients, and those efforts should be more than token. He went on to testify that nothing in the regulations requires "aggressive" collection activities. If hospitals wish to offer discounts from customary charges in connection with a charity-care policy, they may do so as long as they report the full charge for the service on applicable Medicare cost reports. Finally, although conceding that the calculation of the

Medicare and Medicaid disproportionate share payments does not include consideration of uncompensated care, Kuhn stated that these payments to select hospitals amounted to CMS doing its share "to reimburse hospitals for the treatment of uninsured individuals."

EMTALA

The lawsuits also implicate other legal issues unrelated to the charity-care requirements. In 1986, the government enacted EMTALA.[15] A few years later, the government amended EMTALA to add a provision that precluded Medicare-participating hospitals from delaying a medical screening examination or stabilizing treatment to inquire about a patient's method of payment or insurance status.[16]

EMTALA applies to all Medicare-certified hospitals that operate ERs, whether for-profit or nonprofit.[17] Unlike the tax laws described above, EMTALA contains an explicit, albeit somewhat limited, private right of action. However, that private right of action requires that the plaintiff be injured as a result of a hospital's violation of EMTALA.

Knowing what information is public

The class action complaints referenced above routinely refer to three primary information sources in compiling the factual allegations against hospitals:

1. The hospital or system's Form 990
2. Organizational Web sites
3. Annual reports

The law requires that exempt organizations make up to the three most recent Form 990s, or information returns, filed with the IRS (without Schedule B) available to anyone who requests it within periods prescribed by IRS regulations. In addition, an organization known as GuideStar maintains a Web-accessible database about public charities that includes, in most cases, copies of the organizations' Forms 990. The Form 990 provides a wealth of operational and financial information concerning the filing entity. Hospitals and health systems often do a poor job using their 990s to educate the public with respect to how much of their revenue is dedicated to programs that benefit the public, such as wellness programming, community education, and free or low-cost screenings.

Many of the class-action complaints have quoted verbatim content from the defendant hospitals' Web sites claiming charity-care and community benefits. Similarly, many complaints contain references to the defendant organization's annual report, which is often included on organizational Web sites.

A fourth source of information is of significant importance. When a hospital files a collection action against a patient to collect amounts owed to the hospital for care provided, the lawsuit and all of the documents filed in connection with the action become public information. Two phenomena have resulted from the class-action litigation described above. First, counsel across the country are using the Scruggs' theory of unconscionable contract (i.e., charging the uninsured full charges while offering discounts to insurers) as an affirmative defense to collection actions. Second, collection efforts are being utilized by the Scruggs' legal consortium to recruit class representatives.

Summary

The effect of the class-action litigation and congressional and government agency attention on the hospital industry is far reaching, not only for those hospitals targeted for lawsuits but also for those that are not. Although Congress seems temporarily appeased by the AHA's adoption of a Statement of Principles and Guidelines for Hospital Billing and Collection Practices, there is no guarantee that Congress will not take legislative action regarding a perceived public issue. Hospitals and health systems should examine their public filings, charity care/financial assistance policies and processes, debt collection contracts, policies and procedures, and EMTALA compliance policies and procedures to assess their potential exposure and to make changes designed to address some of the more salient issues arising out of the class action litigation. Although an organization obviously cannot change the past, it can gather documentation in support of its previously established practices and filed reports. In light of public sentiment, recent regulatory interpretations, propaganda issued in connection with the class-action litigation, and Congressional review, hospitals should consider modifying their charity-care documents and practices.

Notes

1. Plaintiffs' counsel reportedly received $874 million in legal fees from the tobacco litigation settlements.

2. *www.nfplitigation.com*

3. Himmelstein, David U.; Warren, Elizabeth; Thorne, Deborah; and Woolhandler, Steffie; Health Affairs, "MarketWatch: Illness And Injury As Contributors To Bankruptcy," *The Policy Journal of the Health Sphere* (February 2, 2005).

4. Rev. Rul. 56-185, 1956-1 C.B. 202 (1956).

5. Rev. Rul. 69-545, 1969-2 CB 117 (1969).

6. Eastern Kentucky Welfare Rights Organization v. Simon, 506 F.2d 1278 (D.C. Cir. 1974). The U.S. Supreme Court ruled that the plaintiffs in the action did not suffer an injury and lacked standing to bring suit, thereby setting the groundwork for the long-standing nature of the ruling. The Supreme Court's ruling in the Eastern Kentucky case will likely become central to the defenses mounted by the hospitals and health systems named in the class action lawsuits.

7. Sound Health Association v. Commission, 71 T.C. 158 (1978); Harding Hospital, Inc. v. United States, 505 F.2d 1068 (6th Cir. 1974).

8. IRS Field Service Advice 200110030 (February 5, 2001).

9. *www.dhhs.gov/news/press/2004pres.20040219.html*.

10. 42 U.S.C. §1320a-7b(b).

11. This exclusion authority becomes less of an issue as the programs move almost entirely away from cost or charge-based reimbursement toward across the board prospective payment systems.

12. 68 *FR* 58939.

13. The applicable safe harbor applies to hospital inpatient services that are reimbursable under PPS. One of the requirements for taking advantage of the safe harbor is that the hospital not report the foregone amount as bad debt pursuant to Medicare or Medicaid bad debt rules as described below.

14. Medicare requires that in order for bad debt (limited to uncollectible copays and deductibles from Medicare beneficiaries for covered services) to be included on a hospital's cost report, the hospital must utilize reasonable collection efforts comparable to the effort applied to non-Medicare patients. 42 CFR. §413.80; Medicare Provider Reimbursement Manual, Transmittal 5 (Sept. 12, 2003). Medicare guidance goes so far as to require that the provider issue bills, collection letters, and telephone calls or personal contacts to demonstrate genuine efforts, and if non-Medicare accounts are referred to collection agencies, Medicare accounts must be similarly referred. Transmittal 5 @ 11-11.

15. 42 U.S.C. §1395dd.

16. 42 U.S.C. §1395dd(h).

17. It would be understandable if Congress reevaluated the prong of the IRS' community benefit standard that relies on the provision of emergency medical services without regard to a patient's ability to pay as being sufficient to establish charitability in light of the application of EMTALA's almost identical requirements to both for-profit and tax-exempt hospitals.

Accounting principles and state programs

Accounting principles and state programs

Applicable accounting principles

Originally, the financial accounting and reporting guidelines for bad debts and charity did not require separate reporting. In 1978, the Healthcare Financial Management Association's (HFMA) Principles and Practices Board issued Statement Number 2. Although this statement acknowledged that there was a valid basis for differentiating between charity and bad debts, it determined that the accounting and reporting for these services were the same. Thus, throughout the 1980s, it was difficult to distinguish between these two types of accounts and accurately identify the amounts of each type of uncompensated care provided to patients.

In 1990, after review and approval by the Financial Accounting Standards Board, the American Institute of Certified Public Accountants (AICPA) published a new healthcare accounting guide titled *Audits of Providers of Health Care Services*. Although the AICPA revised the guide in 1996, it made no changes to the sections relating to bad debt and charity care. In response, in 1993, HFMA's Principles and Practices Board issued Statement Number 15, *Valuation and Financial Statement Presentation of Charity Service and Bad Debts by Institutional Healthcare Providers*.[1] HFMA completed a technical update of this document in 1997 to ensure conformity with the technical references in the 1996 AICPA update. The Internal Revenue Service has recognized Statement Number 15 as the prevailing guidance for all reporting of charity care in healthcare institutions.

We have based the following sections on the contents of Statement Number 15. They form the basis for the provider treatment and reporting rules.

Accounting principles for charity care

Healthcare providers are required to distinguish charity care from bad debt expense. By uniformly applying the requirements of Statement Number 15, providers enable the users of their financial statements to make valid comparisons of financial information.

Charity-care background

Charity is different from bad debts. Bad debts occur when the patient is unwilling to pay for the services provided, whereas charity results from a proven inability to pay. This difference is important for the following reasons:

- Charity service represents the consumption of valuable resources that must be managed wisely

- Charity service is one of the important indicators of the fulfillment of an organization's charitable purposes and, therefore, should be clearly identified and disclosed

- Provider eligibility for certain financial assistance is dependent on identification of charity service

- Bad debt expense is a measure of the effectiveness of the organization's credit and collection process[2]

The government requires all types of healthcare providers (e.g., tax-exempt, for-profit, and governmental) to separate bad debts from charity services. The guidelines require providers to classify bad debts as an expense. Organizations must eliminate charity-care dollars from both revenue and receivables. Finally, each provider is required to disclose its charity policy and the amount of charity care it provided. However, the government leaves the extent of the disclosure and the composition of the total amount classified as charity care/community service to the discretion of each provider.

The guidelines also recognize that the type of credit provided to healthcare customers is substantially different from the credit provided in a typical sales situation. Thus, the facility may provide needed healthcare services regardless of the patient's ability to pay. Each organization needs to take into account the financial status of each patient, the cost of bad debts, the time to collect accounts, and overall management of receivables when setting bad debt and charity policies.

Criteria for charity care

Each healthcare provider establishes its charity-care policy and procedures so they are consistent with the facility's mission and values. If the provider has financial resources designated for charity care, such as a trust fund, that provider's policy and dollar limitations may be very different from those of a provider who must recover the cost of charity services from general operations.

Available community/state resources also influence charity policies. Government programs impose criteria for eligibility for charity assistance. However, the provider is not obligated to use these external criteria when developing internal charity criteria.

There is no all-inclusive list of factors that providers must use to develop charity-care criteria. However, the following factors are generally considered to be important components of a charity determination:

- Individual or family income

- Individual or family net worth

- Employment status and earning capacity

- Family size

- Other financial obligations

- The amount and frequency of bills for healthcare services

- Other sources of payment for the services rendered[3]

Statement Number 15 does not mandate the use of a specific guideline for income eligibility determinations. The most common basis for using individual or family income in charity determinations is some derivative of the federal poverty guidelines (FPG), which the Department of Health and Human Services updates annually. Providers typically set the eligibility level at the base guideline amount, or some percentage thereof. For example, a provider may elect to use a sliding scale based at 200% of the current FPG (Figure 3.1).

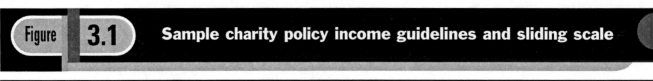

Figure 3.1   Sample charity policy income guidelines and sliding scale

Family Size	Income Guideline (Based at 200% of FPG)	Range 100% W/O	Range 90%	Rannge 80%	Range 70%	Range 60%	Range 50%	Range 40%	Range 30%	Range 20%	Range 10%	No W/O
1	$19,140	$0	$21,054	$22,968	$24,882	$26,796	$28,710	$30,624	$32,538	$34,452	$36,366	
		$19,140	$19,141	$21,055	$22,969	$24,883	$26,797	$28,711	$30,625	$32,539	$34,453	$36,367
2	$25,660	$0	$28,226	$30,792	$33,358	$35,924	$38,490	$41,056	$43,622	$46,188	$48,754	
		$25,660	$25,661	$28,227	$30,793	$33,359	$35,925	$38,491	$41,057	$43,623	$46,189	$48,755
3	$32,180	$0	$35,398	$38,616	$41,834	$45,052	$48,270	$51,488	$54,706	$57,924	$61,142	
		$32,180	$32,181	$35,399	$38,617	$41,835	$45,053	$48,271	$51,489	$54,707	$57,925	$61,143
4	$38,700	$0	$42,570	$46,440	$50,310	$54,180	$58,050	$61,920	$65,790	$69,660	$73,530	
		$38,700	$38,701	$42,571	$46,441	$50,311	$54,181	$58,051	$61,921	$65,791	$69,661	$73,531
5	$45,220	$0	$49,742	$54,264	$58,786	$63,308	$67,830	$72,352	$76,874	$81,396	$85,918	
		$45,220	$45,221	$49,743	$54,265	$58,787	$63,309	$67,831	$72,353	$76,875	$81,397	$85,919
6	$51,740	$0	$56,914	$62,088	$67,262	$72,436	$77,610	$82,784	$87,958	$93,132	$98,306	
		$51,740	$51,741	$56,915	$62,089	$67,263	$72,437	$77,611	$82,785	$87,959	$93,133	$98,307
7	$58,260	$0	$64,086	$69,912	$75,738	$81,564	$87,390	$93,216	$99,042	$104,868	$110,694	
		$58,260	$58,261	$64,087	$69,913	$75,739	$81,565	$87,391	$93,217	$99,043	$104,869	$110,695
8	$64,780	$0	$71,258	$77,736	$84,214	$90,692	$97,170	$103,648	$110,126	$116,604	$123,082	
		$64,780	$64,781	$71,259	$77,737	$84,215	$90,693	$97,171	$103,649	$110,127	$116,605	$123,083
9	$71,300	$0	$78,430	$85,560	$92,690	$99,820	$106,950	$114,080	$121,210	$128,340	$135,470	
		$71,300	$71,301	$78,431	$85,561	$92,691	$99,821	$106,951	$114,081	$121,211	$128,341	$135,471
10	$77,820	$0	$85,602	$93,384	$101,166	$108,948	$116,730	$124,512	$132,294	$140,076	$147,858	
		$77,820	$77,821	$85,603	$93,385	$101,167	$108,949	$116,731	$124,513	$132,295	$140,077	$147,859
11	$84,340	$0	$92,774	$101,208	$109,642	$118,076	$126,510	$134,944	$143,378	$151,812	$160,246	
		$84,340	$84,341	$92,775	$101,209	$109,643	$118,077	$126,511	$134,945	$143,379	$151,813	$160,247
12	$90,860	$0	$99,946	$109,032	$118,118	$127,204	$136,290	$145,376	$154,462	$163,548	$172,634	
		$90,860	$90,861	$99,947	$109,033	$118,119	$127,205	$136,291	$145,377	$154,463	$163,549	$172,635

For family units with more than 12 members, add $6,520 for each additional member; use different base for Alaska and Hawaii.

Breakdown of charity-care criteria

Statement Number 15 recognizes the following charity-care criteria:

Net worth is typically defined as all liquid and nonliquid assets owned, minus all liabilities owed. However, in recent years, many providers have modified this classic definition to exclude the debtor's primary residence. Other exclusions may include retirement funds, student funds, etc.

Employment status speaks to the guarantor's earning capacity and the likelihood that future earnings will be adequate to resolve the healthcare debt within a set period of time. For example, if a provider extends a payment-plan term for a maximum of 12 months, then the guarantor's wages would need to be sufficient to make reasonable monthly payments to resolve the debt within the 12-month period. Otherwise, the earnings would not disqualify the guarantor for charity consideration.

The FPG also consider *family size,* which includes all familial residents of the household. Likewise, the government uses the income of all individuals in the family when applying the FPG amounts to the eligibility determination.

Statement Number 15 does not define other financial obligations, other than to include *living expenses* and other items that are reasonable and necessary. Providers need to determine what items to include in this category. Examples include mortgage(s), loans, credit cards and charge account balances, rent, utilities, food, over-the-counter and prescription drugs, clothing, education costs, etc.

Medical bills are a separate category of expenses. Although providers base the patient's eligibility for charity care on factors present at the time of service, they may also consider past and likely future needs. Within this context, providers may establish criteria for catastrophic medical care and a medically indigent status.

How to apply charity-care criteria

Statement Number 15 contains a caution to providers. Specifically, it advises providers to avoid using rigid criteria. Because a number of factors are involved in making an appropriate charity determination, staff should have the flexibility to apply sound judgment to each case.

Providers are free to apply similar criteria in different ways. For example, one provider may establish a procedure to deem certain types of cases as automatically qualified for charity, while another provider may require case-by-case determinations. Likewise, a provider may define medical indigence as a patient covered by Medicare and Medicaid and may allow charity processing based on the validity of this insurance coverage. Another provider may opt to require completed charity applications for this class of patients.

A similar situation exists in relationship to convertible/liquid assets, the patient's net worth, and a catastrophic medical situation. One provider may require that the patient apply a percentage of his or her assets to the outstanding medical bills, whereas another provider may execute the charity determination based on the catastrophic nature of the medical expenses.

Providers must also discuss two other issues regarding the criteria used to make charity determinations:

- The availability of the information
- The verification of the information

The provider's procedures for charity-care determinations should also discuss how to process applications when the provider cannot determine eligibility for charity care due to insufficient information. Likewise, providers should base the verification process on the material value involved. For example, it is not sound business practice to expend four hours of staff time to verify eligibility for a $50 charity adjustment. Conversely, it is well worth spending four hours to determine charity eligibility for a patient with a bill of $35,000. The provider should identify the verification steps required to provide a cost-effective process.

Note: Base the amount of charity on the amount due after all other resources are applied. This means that providers can apply charity to balances after insurance payments. However, review the terms of each payer contract to avoid a violation relating to collection of amounts due after insurance payment.

Timing of charity-care determinations

There is no set rule as to when organizations should complete determinations of eligibility for charity care. It is acceptable to complete the determination before, during, or after the completion of the service. The availability of information and the degree of verification needed will affect the timing of the charity processing.

Collection activities may also provide information about a patient's eligibility for charity service. Facilities may make eligibility determinations during any phase of the collection process, including during pursuit of accounts by outside collection agencies.

One timing issue is clearly defined in Statement Number 15. Specifically, the statement says "eligibility for charity service relates to fulfilling the provider's criteria when service is rendered."[4] Thus, subsequent events do not impact the charity determination. For example, a patient who was employed at the time of service and, therefore, agreeable to a payment plan does not suddenly become eligible for charity for that occasion of service if the patient is now unemployed.

Also, a provider should not reverse an appropriate charity determination because the patient subsequently obtained a financial windfall. However, providers should use any information that more accurately describes the patient's financial situation at the time of service in the eligibility determination. Providers may correct erroneous determinations, but accounting principles do not permit wholesale reclassification of bad debts to charity or vice versa.

Recording charity-care services

Organizations do not report charity service in revenue or receivables. The practical application of this tenant, however, requires the use of a charity-care provision and allowance, because the provider will not usually have completed the charity determination at the time of service. This concept is the same one that is used for the recording and tracking of bad debts.

Thus, organizations record charges at the gross amount. When the charity determination is processed, the organization posts the adjustments to revenue and accounts receivable through the patient accounting system. Each month, the organization should adjust its allowance for charity services and provisions for charity service accounts to ensure adequate reserves for charity service provided but not yet identified and recorded.

Although Statement Number 15 does not specifically address this issue, providers should maintain records related to the amounts of charity care provided. These records should be in an auditable form to allow for validation of the amount of charity care provided.

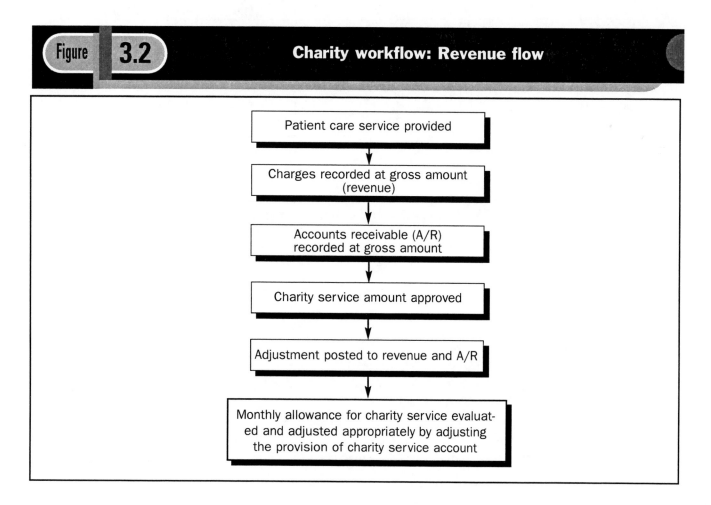

Figure 3.2 — Charity workflow: Revenue flow

Patient care service provided

↓

Charges recorded at gross amount (revenue)

↓

Accounts receivable (A/R) recorded at gross amount

↓

Charity service amount approved

↓

Adjustment posted to revenue and A/R

↓

Monthly allowance for charity service evaluated and adjusted appropriately by adjusting the provision of charity service account

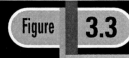

Sample accounting entries

Daily entry:

Detail	Debit	Credit
Patient service provided:		
Accounts receivable	$1,000	
Patient service revenue		$1,000
-to record patient services provided		
Charity application approved:		
Deduction from revenue (charity deduction)	$500	
Accounts receivable		$500
-to record approval of 50% discount for charity		

Month-end entry:

Detail	Debit	Credit
Month end adjustments:		
Provision for charity service (contra revenue account)	$250,600	
Allowance for charity service (receivable contra account)		$250,600
-to record month-end charity adjustment based on A/R analysis		

Note: The details of the month-end analysis and the formula(s) used to develop the amount of the adjustment will vary from facility to facility. In general, this adjustment is an estimate of the outstanding charity service that will be applied to the stated accounts receivable. The result is to reduce revenue and accounts receivable to the appropriate net amounts.

Valuation and disclosure of charity care

Providers initially record charity care as gross charges. For external financial statements, the organization reduces patient accounts receivable by the allowance for charity care, and reduces patient service revenues by the provision for charity care. This process results in a lack of charity-care information clearly stated within the operating statement. A provider may elect to include information about charity care on the face of the operating statement; however, Statement Number 15 makes it clear that "such disclosure should generally be limited to a reference to the note that discusses the provision of charity service."[5]

More commonly, providers disclose charity care in one or several of the following notes to the financial statements:

- A note in the operating statement

- A note disclosing the provider's charity policy (this is required)

- A note disclosing the amount of charity provided based on charges

- A note disclosing the amount of charity provided based on cost

- A note disclosing the amount of charity care provided based on units of service or other statistical information

According to Statement Number 15, HFMA's principles and practice board recommends a single note that encompasses a description of the provider's charity policy, the volume or amount provided, receipts relating to charity care, and disclosure of payment shortfalls (optional). The provider's auditors and internal financial management professionals determine the exact wording and placement of the note(s).

What does this mean for the patient financial services (PFS) department? It means that PFS should take care to correctly process and document the amount of charity care provided. The organization should review the PFS department's recordkeeping and adjustment process annually in conjunction with the annual audit. By engaging in a dialog with the provider's audit team and finance department management, PFS management can ensure the timely and accurate reporting of charity care.

State laws and programs

The following discussion of state laws and programs is current as of January 2005. We do not mean this to be an all-inclusive and comprehensive presentation of state programs—rather, it provides a basic understanding of the kinds of state programs currently in place. Readers should check with their state hospital association for additional information.

Tax-exemption status by state

There is a public presumption that tax emption under Section 501(c)(3) of the Internal Revenue Code automatically qualifies a provider for tax-exempt status under state law. However, each state's constitution and statutory provisions determine state law tax exemption status. Why is this distinction important? For healthcare providers, the issue is exemption from property and other taxes levied at the state level. If the provider meets the criteria to be a charity and it uses its property to further its charitable purpose, then the tax exemption is worth significant dollars.

Each state has specific laws governing tax exemptions, but there are several common themes:

- The provider must be organized as a not-for-profit under the laws of the state, and it must list a charitable purpose in its articles of incorporation

- The provider must receive charitable contributions, which, for most providers, are handled through the provider's foundation

- The provider must provide free care, a benefit to persons, and services that otherwise would need to be provided by the government

- The provider's profits must not benefit individuals, only the provider organization as a whole

State court cases have focused not on the charitable purpose issue, but on the billing and collection practices of providers. Typically, other than advertising the availability of Hill-Burton Funds (a federal program through which hospitals obtain funds in return for providing community service through free care) during the 1980s, many providers have not, until recently, promoted the availability of free or charity care. Providers have clarified their obligations under the Emergency Medical Treatment and Labor Act regulations to provide emergency care to all individuals, regardless of the patient's ability to pay, but beyond the emergency care issues, charity has often been viewed as a payer of last resort.

As previously discussed, because the definition of charity care is not standardized, it is subject to disagreements as state taxing authorities and providers seek to determine the amounts of charity care provided. In addition to determining *what* constitutes charity care, there is the related issue of how to establish the *value* of charity care. Did the provider base patient-care dollars on costs or charges? If the facility uses shortfalls from Medicare or Medicaid, does it base these shortfalls on costs or on charges? Providers need to answer these questions as part of their disclosure process.

Specific state legislative initiatives in 2004

Throughout 2004, several state legislatures attempted to enact legislation governing hospital business practices and charity care. The proposed legislation in Alabama (HB 805) would have limited charges to uninsured individuals to the Medicare payment rates. In Illinois, SB 2579 tried to force hospitals to develop programs to assist the uninsured and to set limits on collection activities. The California legislature actually passed (and the governor vetoed) SB 379, which would have required the provision of discounted care to low-income patients and prohibited aggressive collection techniques. In its place, California hospitals have pledged to comply with the California Healthcare Association's voluntary guidelines. Finally, the Georgia legislature introduced two bills that would have limited charges to uninsured patients to the average rate charged to managed care plans.

All the state legislative initiatives about charity care focused on eliminating the aggressive collection techniques used by some hospitals and ensuring that appropriate discounting programs are in place.

The Washington state example

The state of Washington enacted charity-care legislation, effective July 1, 1989, long before many legislators focused on this issue. Under this legislation, patients may qualify for charity care based on income and resources. Any private healthcare insurance or government program(s) for which the patient qualifies must also pay their share before the charity program applies.

Washington determines charity eligibility based on three levels of income and resources:

- Income at or below 100% of the FPG, adjusted for family size, qualifies for 100% free care. No resource limitations apply.

- Income between 100% and 200% of the FPG, adjusted for family size, qualifies for discounted care based on a sliding scale established by each hospital. The hospital has the option to impose a resource limitation.

- Income above 200% of the FPG, adjusted for family size, may be eligible for a discount if their resources are not sufficient to allow payment of the hospital charges. Hospitals determine whether to reduce charges at this level.

Hospitals are free to enact charity rules more generous than those provided by these guidelines.

Washington hospitals must post or openly display in public areas information concerning the availability of charity and discounted care. During the registration process, hospitals are required to provide patients with written and verbal instructions concerning the charity-care application process. Once the application is completed, there is a two-part determination process. The initial determination, based on verbal information, halts collection and deposit activity. Thereafter, the patient has at least 14 days to provide the required documentation to enable the hospital to make the final charity determination. Hospitals are not allowed to require so much information that patients are discouraged from applying for charity care. Once the hospital receives the documentation, it has 14 days to render its decision on the charity request.

The Washington statute also requires that hospitals provide a denial notice and, if the patient's income is less than 200% of the FPG, notify the patient that he or she may appeal the decision. The patient has 30 days to initiate the appeal process. Once the patient files the appeal, the facility may not pursue collection activity until the appeal is resolved. If the provider denies the appeal, it must notify the patient and the department of health. Thus, the state reviews all charity denials to ensure that providers do not inappropriately deny charity care.

The hospitals are required to make charity determinations in a timely manner; however, at any time upon discovering that the patient may qualify for charity, the hospital is obligated to pursue the charity determination. Patients may pursue charity denials through the department of health and through the court system.

The Washington legislation is an example of what may occur in more states unless hospitals voluntarily adopt reasonable billing and collection practices.

Disproportionate share hospital funds: State pools

Sixteen states have approved programs for meeting the federal requirements to provide additional payments to hospitals that provide a disproportionate share of uncompensated care to the indigent and uninsured.

Typically, the state levies provider assessments against all hospitals to generate the funding for this program. States then pool the assessment dollars with matching federal Medicaid disproportionate share hospital (DSH) funds. The state then distributes the total pool of funds back to the hospitals using a preestablished formula involving Medicaid costs and uncompensated care costs. The federal government requires that the assessment rate be uniform for all providers and that 10% of the hospitals receive less than their assessed amounts in funding from the pooled fund. Detailed program rules, including distribution schedules, recordkeeping requirements, and eligibility rules, are state-specific. However, before hospitals implement them, the Centers for Medicare & Medicaid Services (CMS) must approve the program.

Why is understanding this type of funding important to a discussion of charity or uncompensated care? First, specific recordkeeping, logs, patient applications, eligibility rules, and timing of income validation impose very detailed requirements on PFS staff. Second, these state pool programs have a direct impact on each provider's charity-care policies and procedures. Finally, for non-pool state providers, the program eligibility requirements and application procedures may be useful for developing individual charity care policies and procedures.

A pooled funds state example: The state of Ohio

The Hospital Care Assurance Program (HCAP) in Ohio is an example of a CMS-approved funds program. Since 1987, Ohio hospitals have participated in this program, which Subchapter XIX of the Social Security Act of 1945, specifically at 42 U.S.C. Sec. 1396r-4, governs. In 1992, Ohio enacted the "Free Care Requirement" law, which requires hospitals to provide basic, medically necessary services regardless of the patient's ability to pay. Specifically, hospitals must provide free care to any Ohio resident whose family income is less than the FPG at the time of service. Annually, the state enacts and provides all Ohio hospitals with program administration rules governing definitions of DSH, the assessment structure, and the distribution formula. Payment and distributions occur on a schedule that the state publishes annually.

The HCAP rules require Ohio providers to post signs and notices concerning the HCAP program in their emergency room, all admission areas, and all places where patients pay their bills. Requirements for the notice include the following:

- The notices must inform eligible individuals of their right to receive basic, medically necessary hospital services without charge

- The text must be clear and use simple terms that the average person in the service area can understand

- Notices must be printed in English and any other language(s) common to the provider's service area

- The notice must be legible from a distance of 20 feet or from the expected distance patients will stand from the sign

- Providers must make reasonable efforts to communicate the content of the posted notice to individuals who cannot read

Specific billing requirements are associated with the HCAP program. Hospitals must include notification about the HCAP program with at least the first and second hospital bill. Information to be provided includes the following:

- An explanation that individuals whose income is at or below the FPG are able to obtain medically necessary hospital services at no charge

- The specific levels of the FPGs at the time of billing

- The process for applying for free care under the HCAP program

The state of Ohio specifically discourages the use of the term "HCAP" in the billing notices. Hospitals must use terms such as "free care" or services "free of charge." In addition, as of December 12, 2000, hospitals must reference the HCAP notice on the front of the hospital bill or statement.

There is no mandated application form for the HCAP application. However, the Ohio Hospital Association and the Ohio Department of Job and Family Services (ODJFS) provide a recommended application form that contains all the data elements needed to comply with the HCAP eligibility determination rules.

Figure	3.4	ODJFS sample application for HCAP

PATIENT NAME: _____ DATE OF APPLICATION: _____

APPLICANT NAME, IF NOT PATIENT: _____
(If the applicant is not the patient, please answer the following questions as they apply to the patient.)

STREET: _____ CITY: _____

STATE:_____ ZIP CODE: _____

DATE(S) OF HOSPITAL SERVICE: From _____ To _____
Were you an Ohio resident at the time of
your hospital service?   Yes____ No____

Were you an active Medicaid recipient at the time
of your hospital service?   Yes____ No____
If yes, Medicaid recipient ID number: _____

Were you an active recipient of Disability
Assistance at the time of your hospital service?   Yes ____ No____
(If you answered Yes to this question, please attach a copy of your
DA card effective during your hospital service to this application.)

Did you have health insurance (other than
Medicaid) at the time of your hospital service?   Yes____ No____

Please provide the following information for all of the people in your immediate family who live in your
home. For purposes of HCAP, "family" is defined as the patient, the patient's spouse, and all of the
patient's children under 18 (natural or adoptive) who live in the patient's home.

Name	Age	Relationship to patient	Income for three months prior to hospital service*	Income for 12 months prior to hospital service*	Type of income verification attached**
(Patient)		self			
Total persons in family		**Total family income**			

*Income verification must accompany this application. If you reported $0 income provide a brief
explanation on the back of this form or on an attached sheet.
**Income verification may include income tax returns, pay stubs, w-2s, or other documents containing
income information for the appropriate time period (three or 12 months prior to hospital service).

**By my signature below, I certify that everything I have stated on this application and on any
attachments is true.**

_____   _____
Applicant Signature   Date

Source: Ohio Hospital Association. Reprinted with permission.

The eligibility requirements linked to income and family size are the sole criteria required by the program. Note that the program requires both three-month and 12-month calculations, and the hospital is required to use whichever calculation most benefits the patient. Thus, there is no requirement to consider other assets in making the eligibility determination. This clause is different than the multiple criteria recommended by both Statement Number 15 and the Medicare program recommendations for discounting charges.

There is a three-year limit for applying for free care for dates of service on or after December 14, 2000. If the hospital cannot verify the patient's income or family size on the date of service, the application does not qualify for HCAP.

Hospitals may choose to require that the patient first apply for Medicaid before processing the HCAP application. However, hospitals don't have to require a Medicaid application. Likewise, hospitals should pursue liability coverage; however, the hospital does not have to prove that liability coverage does not exist in order to process the HCAP application.

Ohio hospitals are required to have written policies and procedures for charity care that detail the application process and the kinds of materials required to establish income and family size. Auditors use these procedures to validate amounts reported on the Ohio Medicaid cost report forms.

The audit process includes four documentation reviews for each of the randomly selected facilities. The state auditors complete a medical record review to ensure compliance with documentation requirements for the date(s) of service written off to the program. The eligibility determination review validates that the facilities followed the eligibility criteria and excluded other insurance amounts from the HCAP write-offs. The policy and procedures review includes compliance with state law, as well as consistency, disability assistance, income and family determination practices, notifications, billing, and the application form used by the provider.

The financial records and reporting requirements for HCAP include a separate schedule (Schedule F) on the Ohio Medicaid cost report and the supporting detailed logs of accounts written off to the program. The log requirements include

• all uncompensated care accounts for patients in the disability assistance program

- all uncompensated care accounts for patients with income below 100% of the poverty level (UC<100%)

- all uncompensated care accounts for patients with income greater than 100% of the poverty level (UC>100%), segregated by inpatient accounts with and without insurance and outpatient accounts with and without insurance

Data requirements for all logs include patient name, patient account number, date of service, date of write-off, total charges, and amount written off to HCAP. Only medically necessary hospital charges can be included in the amounts claimed on the logs. In addition, Ohio hospitals cannot claim an account as both a Medicare bad debt and an HCAP account. CMS has ruled that once the patient applies for and the facility grants HCAP approval, there is no patient liability and, therefore, no Medicare bad debt.

As this summary of program content indicates, the pooled funds program imposes considerable record-keeping and reporting requirements on hospital PFS departments. However, without these pooled funds programs, millions of federal DSH dollars would not be available to hospitals in the pooled funds states.

States using the American Hospital Association (AHA) guidelines

The states of California, Florida, Illinois, Minnesota, New York, Oregon, Pennsylvania, Tennessee, and Wisconsin have developed and publicized documents outlining the principles and guidelines for assisting low-income and uninsured patients with healthcare services. The states based the principles and guidelines statements on the "Hospital Billing and Collection Practices" statement produced by the board of trustees of the AHA. This statement calls upon hospitals to

- treat all patients equitably, with dignity, with respect, and with compassion

- serve the emergency healthcare needs of everyone, regardless of a patient's ability to pay for care

- assist patients who cannot pay for part or all of the care they receive

- balance needed financial assistance for some patients with broader fiscal responsibilities in order to keep hospitals' doors open for all who may need care in a community[6]

There are five sections to the AHA's guidelines. First, the guidelines call upon hospitals to communicate effectively with patients. This includes providing financial counseling and publicizing the availability of the financial counseling service. Hospitals should use a billing process that can be readily understood by the patient. If a patient inquiry is received, the hospital should respond promptly. Finally, hospitals need to communicate meaningful information concerning charges for available services.

Second, patients often do not know or understand hospital billing practices. Therefore, hospitals need to provide customer-friendly information concerning their charity and financial assistance programs. This information should be available to everyone in the community. Also, hospitals should write policies and procedures in easy-to-understand terms and make these policies and procedures available to other community agencies that assist individuals in need.

Third, hospitals need to consistently and accurately apply the policies and procedures developed in support of charity care and financial assistance. Training for all staff who may become involved in patient inquiries concerning charity care and financial assistance is important. This includes not only PFS staff but also nurses, social workers, etc.

Fourth, the AHA guidelines urge hospitals to make care affordable to individuals with limited means by ensuring that charges are reasonable. It encourages discount policies, even for individuals who do not qualify for charity care (either wholly or in part). This guideline also encourages providers to clearly indicate eligibility criteria, discount amounts, and payment plan options.

Finally, the AHA guidelines encourage hospitals to develop fair billing and collection practices. Collection activities pursued both internally and by external collection agencies should be within a clearly defined scope of practice. Policies for collection of accounts should be written with authority (approval levels) included in the procedures.

The guidelines also recognize that individual state statutes and regulations may necessitate a modification to the guidelines, to the extent necessary to comply with state requirements.

As of January 3, 2005, the AHA reported that more than 3,900 hospitals nationwide had agreed to the AHA "Hospital Billing and Collection Practices" statement.

Differences between state guidelines

Although the state associations used the AHA statement as a starting point, there are differences among the state guidelines. Consider the following examples:

- California sets the recommended poverty level at 300% of the FPG. The guidelines recommend limiting expected patient payments for patients obtaining financial assistance to the Medicare amount, the amount from other government-sponsored programs, or another discounted amount set by the hospital.

- Florida closely copies the AHA statement, which does not suggest an FPG amount. Florida guidelines do not discuss discounting charges.

- Illinois guidelines suggest full charity for income levels up to 100% of the FPG and discounted arrangements for patients with income in the 100%–200% range. Illinois issued its guidelines before the discount clarification letter from Secretary Thompson. Therefore, the guidelines suggest that discounting the patient payment amount from charges may be problematic.

- Minnesota and New York guidelines suggest using the 200% FPG amount and offer options for providers to go above that amount. Both guidelines indicate that discounts from charges are acceptable and that discount practices may differ based on the type of service provided.

- Oregon guidelines call for charity for patients with incomes below 150% of the FPG and a sliding scale and individual consideration for individuals with income above the 150% range. These guidelines suggest the use of sliding scales as the discount mechanism.

- The Pennsylvania guidelines incorporate the AHA guidelines, the Tobacco Settlement Act, and the Institutions of Purely Public Charity Act. The guidelines do not tie specific recommendations to any specific FPG. The guidelines suggest that the hospitals should limit the expected payments from patients obtaining financial assistance to amounts received from any government or contracted payer for the same service.

- Tennessee mirrors the AHA guidelines and includes a sliding scale as the discount mechanism.

- Wisconsin guidelines suggest that individuals below 200% of the FPG should receive charity care. The guidelines suggest either discounting based on a fixed standard (Medicare/Medicaid amounts, commercial contracts, etc.) or using a sliding scale.

All of the state-sponsored guidelines include provisions for written policies and procedures, clear communication with patients, and fair billing and collection practices. The AHA guidelines do not suggest specific details for discounting, only that hospitals should provide such discounts within the scope of federal regulations.

State guidelines for liens and wage garnishment

A final area of interest among the various state guidelines is the issue of liens against the patient's primary residence and garnishment of wages. The AHA statement is silent on these issues.

- California's guidelines clearly suggest that both hospitals and outside collection agencies should not use liens and wage garnishment when dealing with low income, uninsured patients.

- The Florida, Minnesota, and New York guidelines are just the opposite of the California recommendations, but the guidelines do suggest that hospitals should not pursue sale or foreclosure on the patient's primary residence.

- Illinois guidelines permit garnishment of wages but limit the use of liens against the primary residence unless there is sufficient value in the property to suggest that the patient can assume significant financial obligations. The Illinois guidelines do not recommend execution of the lien.

- The Oregon guidelines provide clarification concerning the types of liens available in the state, but are silent as to best practice recommendations.

- Pennsylvania guidelines suggest that hospitals should pursue legal action and liens only when there is evidence that the patient has the ability to pay the outstanding medical bill; the state does not recommend foreclosure on the primary residence.

- Wisconsin recommendations mirror the Pennsylvania guidelines.

Other state initiatives

Information on other state charity practices has been collected from the various state hospital association Web sites. Several states with different types of charity programs are listed in the following section.

Arkansas

The Arkansas Association of Hospital Trustees issued a trustee advisory in the spring of 2004 alerting boards of trustees to their responsibility for ensuring that their organizations "have clear and understandable billing and collection policies that include how hospital costs are itemized on patient bills, policies for charging self-pay patients, financial assistance and charity care policies, and collection procedures."[7] The article also references the HFMA's Patient Friendly Billing project and the AHA guidelines for billing and collection. However, the association has not issued recommended guidelines for Arkansas hospitals.

Colorado

In 1983, the Colorado legislature passed the Colorado Indigent Care Program, which uses state funds to partially reimburse providers, both clinics and hospitals, for services provided to the state's non-Medicaid medically indigent residents. The benefits vary and a network of 49 hospitals, 18 clinics, and 51 satellite facilities provides them. Participating providers are required to prioritize services as follows:

- Emergency care for the entire year

- Additional medical care for conditions deemed the most serious threat to the health of indigent persons

- Any other medical care needs

The program is designed to provide discounted recoveries of the costs of services provided to individuals whose income places them outside the Medicaid program.

New Hampshire

New Hampshire non-profit hospitals are required to perform a community needs assessment once every three years. The state also standardizes the reporting of charity services provided by the hospitals and the reporting of items included in the community benefits provided by each hospital. Charity policies must be available in written form to the public, and hospitals must post the policies in public areas of the facility.

New Hampshire specifically defines charity-care dollars as excluding bad debts. Public health program participation and support are separate, as are other needed community health programs provided to the community by the provider. Donation of funds, property, and services to promote a healthier community is a separate category. Activities related to medical research, as well as education and training of health-care workers, are also separately reported. This act makes New Hampshire a leader in defining for all providers specific categories of reporting for charitable services provided within the state.

New Jersey

New Jersey bases the charity reimbursement amount on the Medicaid prices for the services provided, augmented by the medical education supplements, which are based on the Medicare program formulas. The state individually ranks hospitals based on the relative charity-care percentage, which the state calculates by dividing the hospital's gross patient services charity revenue by the overall patient services gross revenue. The top nine hospitals receive charity-care payments equal to 96% of their hospital-specific documented charity care. The hospital ranked 10th receives two percentage points less in reimbursement, and all ranked lower receive 2% less than the hospital ranked immediately higher, with a lower-end reimbursement rate of 43% of the hospital-specific documented charity care.

Texas

In enacting tort reform, Texas has created an opportunity for hospitals to obtain lower caps for non-economic damage awards (e.g., malpractice suits) by providing significant amounts of charity care. If a hospital qualifies, award limits for malpractice suits are $100,000 instead of the $250,000 limit set in the 1993 law.

Private, nonprofit hospitals qualify for the lower cap by proving that they provide at least 8% of their net patient revenue as charity care. An additional requirement is that the provider must provide at least 40% of the total charity care provided in the county.

Summary

Although the accounting principles and practices related to the classification and reporting of charity-care services are quite specific in many ways, it is still difficult to obtain a comparative picture of the total amount of healthcare services provided to the uninsured and underinsured low income population. As a result, nonprofit healthcare providers face the challenge of defending their tax-exempt status.

All providers participating in state-sponsored charity reimbursement programs face increasingly detailed documentation and logging requirements. Finally, the billing and collection practices within the healthcare industry have come under public and legislative scrutiny, leading many state hospital associations and hospitals to adopt more patient-friendly and economically liberal approaches to the collection of patient accounts.

Notes

1. The full text of Statement No. 15 is located at *www.hfma.org/resource/P_and_P_board/statement_15.htm.*

2. "Principles and Practices Board Statement Number 15," Section 1.4.

3. "Principles and Practices Board Statement Number 15," Section 2.3.

4. "Principles and Practices Board Statement Number 15," Section 3.3.

5. "Principles and Practices Board Statement Number 15," Section 5.3.

6. *www.aha.org/aha/key_issues/bcp/content/guidelinesfinalweb.pdf*

7. *The Arkansas Trusett,* vol. 10, no. 1, (Spring 2004), p. 1.

4

FOUR

Strategies to assess risk and identify opportunities for improvement

Strategies to assess risk and identify opportunities for improvement

As a patient financial services (PFS) professional, how do you know whether you should recommend changes to your facility's current charity process?

No single approach or assessment methodology reveals everything about your charity processes. However, by using different types of data and different survey approaches, it is possible to develop a cohesive picture of your organization's current processes and the opportunities for improvement. You do not need to conduct all of the assessments discussed in this chapter; rather, select the ones that provide you with the most relevant information in a timely manner.

Identify current charity-care processes

There are several general indicators that your organization may have significant issues related to charity care:

1. Your hospital's auditors may have commented on the charity practices as part of the annual audit and management letter. If the audit report included comments related to charity care, you will have until the next audit to address the concerns. Typical concerns in this area focus on the correct classification of write-offs to charity v. bad debt and the availability of supporting documentation for the charity accounts.

2. A review of your customer service contact logs will indicate the volume of contacts concerning charity care and the nature of the calls. A high volume (in the top two to three reasons for contact) of charity calls suggests that patients are not receiving the information they need earlier in the processing cycle.

If your customer service staff is not routinely logging the reason for contacts and regularly providing frequency information, getting started is a simple project. Develop an Excel or Access database with one file per customer service employee. Staff can use a list of call reasons plus "other" to categorize the calls for management use. Examples of reasons for calling include the following:

- To check a balance

- To ask about charity care

- To say they did not receive a service

- To initiate a charity application

- To ask whether insurance was billed

- To find out what a particular test was

- To find out why an account is in collection

- To set up a payment plan

- Other—briefly define

Process reviews

Another way to obtain a snapshot view of current charity processing is to complete the following brief process review with "yes" or "no" responses:

The greater the number of "yes" answers in the pre-service and time-of-service blocks, the more contemporary the charity processes.

| Figure 4.1 | Self survey: Charity processing within the revenue cycle |

Activity	Pre-service process	Time-of-service process	Post-service process
Patient financial education provided concerning charity care			
Charity application form initiated with patient			
Charity application approved or denied			
System generated approval or denial notice produced and mailed			
Adjustment posted			
Appeal process activated			

Note: This worksheet is included on the accompanying CD-ROM.

Any or all of these approaches will provide a generalized view of charity processes and issues. However, with a little effort, you can develop a more detailed analysis of charity processing.

The risk assessment process

The concept of risk assessment is based on developing your hospital-specific data and using that data to identify trends and opportunities. In some cases, regional, state, or national data is used for comparisons. In other cases, you are simply trending your internal performance and using that data to develop performance improvement plans.

Risk assessments fall into several categories:

1. Dollar issues—how much charity and discounted care the organization provides, especially in comparison to geographic peers or national peer groups.

2. Timing of resolution of charity cases.

3. Cost issues—what are the costs of the current process compared to the best practices?

4. Accuracy issues—does the organization correctly process charity applications, is it using payment plans appropriately, or should the organization designate some payment plan accounts as charity accounts?

Risk assessments may take a variety of forms, but an organization can conduct all methods internally or outsource the assessment to a consulting firm. There are advantages and disadvantages associated with both methods.

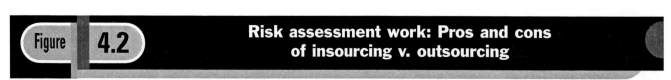

Figure 4.2 Risk assessment work: Pros and cons of insourcing v. outsourcing

Approach	Advantages	Disadvantages
Internal—PFS staff and managers	• No-out-of-pocket expense • Opportunity to examine details as completing work • Understanding of system, notes, etc. • Audit process itself becomes learning experience for staff	• May not apply criteria as rigorously as should be done • Regular work will not be done or overtime will be used to maintain production • May waste time looking at "who" did something instead of following criteria • May have vested interest in results
External—Auditors or consulting firm	• Outside party with no vested interest in results (objectivity issue) • Dedicated staff to complete work in timely manner—no interruptions or distractions from regular work • Experienced in recognizing trends v. outlier situations	• Out-of-pocket costs • Need to schedule and provide work space • Need to learn system and decipher account notes

Regardless of the issue and approach, proper planning and preparation is essential to achieving the desired results. Generally, the following issues need to be considered and resolved before starting the risk assessment:

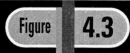

Figure 4.3 — **Specific considerations for internal v. external assessment work by type of assessment**

Category	Internal	External
Dollar issues—Comparison to peers (surveys)	• Identify person to receive responses • Determine what information to gather from the survey • Identify who will create survey instrument(s) and conduct the survey • Define any terms that may be vague in the survey • Identify the survey universe • Identify the survey methodology (e.g., e-mail, letter and form, telephone) • Set time frame for completion of the survey • Identify how samples of materials requested will be received (e.g., mail, e-mail, fax)	• Define approval process for survey instruments • Provide letter introducing consultant to survey targets • Identify the survey universe • Set time frame for completion of the survey
Timeliness of charity resolution	• Determine sample size for project • Select random sample of accounts written off to charity adjustments within the most recent 60-day period; identify the source of accounts • Determine data to be collected (e.g., original financial class, write-off amount, pre-service date, date of service/discharge date, final bill date, charity adjustment date, etc.) • Create data capture tool (worksheet)	• Recommend sample size for project • Select random sample of accounts written off to charity adjustments within the most recent 60-day period; identify source of accounts • Modify data collection tool for specific engagement • Modify database and report formats for specifics of engagement • Obtain system inquiry access and training

Figure 4.3		**Specific considerations for internal v. external assessment work by type of assessment (cont.)**

Category	Internal	External
Timeliness of charity resolution (cont.)	• Create database to record data and summarize results • Identify reports to be graphed from data • Train reviewer(s) on how to collect and record data	
Calculation of costs associated with current processes	• Identify source of costs • Identify costs to be considered	• Identify source of costs • Identify costs to be considered
Confirmation of processing accuracy—Charity applications	• Create sample selection rules • Create data collection tools • Locate files of approved and denied applications • Obtain detailed charity policy and procedures in effect during period included in audit • Create database to record data and summarize results • Train staff on the audit process	• Propose sample selection rules • Modify data collection tools for engagement • Locate files of approved and denied applications • Obtain detailed charity policy and procedures in effect during period included in audit • Open database to record and summarize results • Review application information to understand all data elements
Confirmation of processing accuracy—Charity applications	• Create data collection tools • Create report listing all currently designated payment plan accounts • Obtain detailed payment plan policy and procedures in effect during period included in audit • Create database to record data and summarize results • Train staff on the audit process	• Propose sample selection rules • Modify data collection tools for engagement • Create report listing all currently designated payment plan accounts • Obtain detailed payment plan policy and procedures in effect during the period included in audit • Open database to record and summarize results • Obtain system access and training to review account information online

Source: Sandra J. Wolfskill, FHFMA.

Dollar issues

Risk assessments based on dollar issues may involve several different components. For each component, the group of providers that you compare to your organization should have a geographic and size relationship to the surveying provider. For example, it would not make sense to compare the total charity dollars provided by a 700-bed teaching hospital with those provided by a 50-bed facility. Even if you consider charity dollars as a percentage of net revenue, comparing two facilities of such different sizes may produce distorted results, because the larger institutions typically have a greater ability to absorb charity services. Likewise, comparing charity practices in Alabama with those in New York will produce questionable results. However, it is acceptable to compare within a geographic region, which may span parts or all of several states.

Types of dollar-based comparisons

You can collect dollar-based data and use it to benchmark your organization's performance against a peer group.

First, charity dollars as a percentage of net revenue and bad debt dollars as a percentage of net revenue are standard financial indicators. If a provider reports charity and bad debt as a combined number, don't include that provider in your survey. If your peer group is providing an average of 2.5% of net revenue in charity care and your organization is only providing 1% of its net revenue in charity care, change may be needed.

Another dollar-based comparative relates to the federal poverty guidelines (FPG). Providers typically base their poverty income determination on a percentage of the FPG. The lowest level used is 100% of the FPG. A simple tabulation of the number of providers using 100%, 150%, 200%, 300%, 400%, or other percentage of the FPG allows you to rank your facility against the peer group. Another scale often used is a sliding scale based on some percentage of the FPG table. Identifying whether other providers use a sliding scale (yes/no) and if yes, how the sliding scale is constructed, is also important comparative data.

A third set of dollar data is a comparison of the charity care reported by the nonprofit hospitals on the annual 990 Internal Revenue Service form. However, use this data with caution because not all providers disclose the details of the numbers they report. For example, the total reported may include not only charity dollars, but also bad debts, shortfalls from governmental programs, volunteer hours, community health screenings, etc.—in short, everything that could be classified as uncompensated services.

Surveys

Conducting dollar data surveys is straightforward. The survey should be short and include no more than 10 questions. The actual survey instrument should make it simple for employees to respond and use ranges of data as answers whenever possible.

Defining the universe of hospitals to survey and identifying the appropriate contact person may require more effort. The American Hospital Association directory is a standard source of hospital information, including mailing address and bed size. The Healthcare Financial Management Association (HFMA), National Association of Healthcare Access Managers, and American Association of Health Care Administrative Management membership directories for your area/state readily provide contact information for chief financial officers, patient access directors, and PFS directors. Surveys that include the ability to respond via e-mail are likely to be completed and promptly returned. If your survey uses mail returns, remember to include a stamped, self-addressed envelope with each survey.

What is an acceptable survey response rate? Typically, mailed surveys achieve a 10% response rate; a recent HFMA revenue cycle survey achieved a 22% response rate. Do not expect a 100% response rate, but a rate in the 15%–20% range is acceptable.

How to tabulate results

Begin tabulating survey results as you receive them. Create a simple Excel worksheet and assign the tabulation project to a clerical staff member. For a charity and bad debt as percentage of net revenue survey, a typical spreadsheet would include the information in Figure 4.4.

Figure 4.4	Charity and bad debt provider survey

Provider	Bed size	Charity %	Bad debt %	Date of most recent policy change*
ABC Medical Center	350	2.4%	3.1%	01/01/2004

*Policy change excludes simply updating the FPG scale based on the new federal guidelines published in the spring of each year.

Note: This worksheet is included on the accompanying CD-ROM.

By using a spreadsheet for tabulation, you can perform various data sorts, ranking, mean, and median calculations. Organizations can also create graphic presentations of the data using the Excel graphing features.

Figure 4.5 is an example of the FPG data worksheet:

Figure 4.5	Federal poverty guideline scale survey			
Provider	**Bed size**	**FPG scale used**	**Sliding scale (Y/N)**	**Date of most recent policy change***
ABC Medical Center	350	200%	Y	01/01/2004

*Policy change excludes simply updating the FPG scale based on the new federal guidelines published in February of each year.

Note: This worksheet is included on the accompanying CD-ROM.

Figure 4.6 is an example of the IRS 990 data worksheet:

Figure 4.6	IRS 990 data comparison							
Provider	**Bed size**	**Total $**	**Charity (Y/N)**	**Bad debt (Y/N)**	**C/As (Y/N)**	**Vol Hrs (Y/N)**	**Free health screenings (Y/N)**	**Other (list)**
ABC Medical Center	350	$2.8 million	Y	N	N	Y	Y	None

Note: This worksheet is included on the accompanying CD-ROM.

What is the significance of the dollar-based data comparisons, and what opportunities will comparisons of your performance with that data suggest? Figure 4.7 identifies each type of dollar data and the kinds of opportunities that may be identified from each data source.

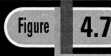

Opportunity data from dollar-based assessments

Dollar data	Opportunity identified
Charity as % of net revenue; bad debt as % of net revenue	Need to increase charity dollars and decrease bad debt dollars
FPG scale percentage used; sliding scale used	Need to increase base of FPG scale used; need to add sliding scale component
IRS Form 990 data	Need to better define data used for preparation of IRS form 990

Note: This worksheet is included on the accompanying CD-ROM.

Process timeliness issues

Risk assessments based on processing timeliness involve establishing when activities occur. A second dimension of the data is the percentage of time when the required activity occurred (i.e., what percentage of the accounts confirmed that a required process activity occurred). For example, if the account represents a scheduled service, was charity screening required and, if so, was it completed in the pre-service timeframe? This data sets the baseline for a provider's internal charity processing standards, which the provider can later compare to results after implementing an improvement project.

Choose the sample

The first step for performing this type of risk assessment involves defining the sample universe and choosing the sample size.

There are two options for defining the *sample universe:*

- If part of the reason for performing the assessment is to determine the overall percentage of encounters qualifying for charity processing, then the approximate universe should include all patients registered in the past 150 days (all registrations approach)

- If your goal is to determine the timeliness of the current process, then the universe should include all charity applications received in a 30- or 60-day period (applications approach)

If you are using the applications approach, be careful to include both approved and denied applications in the sample. Using just the write-offs as the sample source, for example, will not allow the reviewer to document the reasons for application denials.

In either case, the sample selection is a simple random selection.

You can calculate the *sample size* based on statistical parameters or by using a common-sense approach. If you are using the universe of all encounters, it is often best to set a desired confidence factor and use a statistical basis. If you are using all charity applications in a set period, it is acceptable to use the entire universe, unless the number of applications is greater than 400. If the universe is greater than 400 accounts, use random selection to identify approximately 400 accounts. *Note:* Samples greater than 400 accounts entail additional data collection efforts but often do not significantly influence the final results. More information and a calculator to determine sample sizes are available at *www.surveysystem.com/sscalc.htm.*

Set a confidence interval and confidence level

The calculator found at *www.surveysystem.com/sscalc.htm* allows the user to set the confidence interval, which is the plus-or-minus figure reported in most opinion poll results. For example, if the confidence interval is four and 47% percent of the sample produces a specific result, you can be "sure" that if you had sampled the entire universe, between 43% (47-4) and 51% (47+4) would have produced that result.

The confidence level, which organizations state as a percentage, represents how often the true percentage of the universe would produce the result falling within the confidence interval. Typical surveys use either 95% or 99% confidence levels. The 95% confidence level means you can be 95% certain; the 99% confidence level means you can be 99% certain. Using the example cited above, and setting the confidence level at 95%, when you put the confidence level and the confidence interval together, you can say that you are 95% sure that the true percentage of the population is between 43% and 51%.

How to collect the data

Assuming that the assessment focuses only on the timeliness of charity processing, you can use a streamlined worksheet to collect the data. Alternatively, you could directly enter the data into a database application developed for the assessment. If this is a one-time assessment, you can use a simple set of Excel worksheets to produce the results. However, if you will regularly repeat the assessment, then investing in a database application or obtaining such an application from a consulting firm may be the better route to follow.

The purpose of the worksheet is to capture the timeliness of the charity processing from scheduling through final application of the charity adjustment or denial. Concurrently, you can capture the reasons for denied applications for analysis. As the following sample worksheet indicates, capturing timing information and denial information is a matter of reviewing detailed account information from scheduling, registration, and patient accounting systems.

Figure 4.8 — Charity timeliness processing worksheet

Account or ID #				Charity denial codes:
Financial class				1 Eligibility denial
Charity adjustment				2 Incomplete application
Charity denial code				3 Untimely filing
				4 No application received
Key dates: Schedule date	Completed	Incomplete	N/A	5 Other—explain _____
Date of service/discharge				
Final bill date				
Charity adjust/denial date Zero balance date Date initial application Date complete application				

Note: "Not applicable" is used to indicate that the account was not a scheduled service.

Note: This worksheet is included on the accompanying CD-ROM.

Once the data capture is complete, record the elapsed days on an Excel worksheet or in a database file. Ultimately, you should calculate and present averages in a data table or graphic form.

Figure	4.9	Sample data summary

Summary data	Elapsed days			% Occurred—Universe		
	Completed	Incomplete	N/A	Completed	Incomplete	N/A
Sched to DOS	6			60%		40%
DOS to FB	5			100%		
FB to charity adj/denial	85	100		70%	20%	10%
DOS to zero	90			90%	10%	
Sched to charity adj/den	96			55%	5%	40%
DOS to charity adj/den	87	95		85%	15%	
Charity adj/den to zero	31	65		90%	10%	

Denial	% of
Code	15%
Code 2	45%
Code 3	5%
Code 4	30%
Code 5	5%

Sample = 50

Source: Sandra J. Wolfskill, FHFMA.

What does this data indicate? First, there is no pre-service or time of service charity processing; all charity processing is a post-service activity. However, 60% of the accounts were scheduled services, indicating that a significant pre-service opportunity exists. In addition, the primary denial reason is incomplete applications. Opportunities exist to improve application approvals through better instructions, staff assistance in application completion, etc.

This same sample timeliness approach can be used to compare bad debt performance to charity performance by completing a separate review of a similar number of bad debt accounts.

Cost issues

Risk assessments based on the cost of the current process focus on excessive processing costs incurred in a predominately post-service charity-processing model. The details of the assessment will vary from hospital to hospital; however, the following items provide a starting point:

- Statement costs: Production, postage, handling, address forwarding

- Staff costs: Review costs of bad debts to identify potential charity accounts

- Overstatement of days in A/R and/or degraded aging analysis: Cost of impact on bond ratings (interest rates)

This data supplements data obtained through peer surveys and timeliness analyses. Although organizations can achieve hard savings, through a reduction in costs of statements for example, the staffing costs may, in fact, be shifted to achieve charity-processing resolution earlier in the processing cycle. In other words, moving charity processing into the pre-service and time of service parts of the revenue cycle may or may not be work that can be absorbed by existing staff, typically the financial counselors. Therefore, anticipating staffing savings may not be accurate or appropriate.

Figure 4.10	Cost reduction opportunities analysis		
Cost factor	**Cost basis/ source**	**Current costs**	**Future costs if processing shifted to earlier in the revenue cycle**
Statements	Annual costs per statement; # of statements eliminated by process change		
Staff costs	Optional—may not see a reduction in staff costs		
Improvement of A/R— impact on bond ratings	Change in interest expense charged on bonds		
Other—user defined			

Note: This worksheet is included on the accompanying CD-ROM.

Accuracy of charity application processing

Hospitals use audits of charity applications to confirm the accuracy of the charity determinations and adjustments. An additional audit of payment plan accounts identifies missed opportunities to assist patients through charity processing. Audits may be one-time events or organizations may regularly use them as a quality assurance tool for monitoring performance within the PFS department.

Approved charity applications audit

To audit approved charity applications, select a random sample of 50–100 accounts processed within the most recent quarter. Alternatively, select a random sample equal to 20%–25% of all charity applications approved in the most recent quarter. If you would like a statistical basis, use the sample size calculator found at *www.surveysystem.com/sscalc.htm.*

Using a worksheet, capture the following data about each account:

1. Review the eligibility determination against the charity policy and procedures and income guidelines in effect as of the determination date.

2. Trace the approval to the detailed patient account in the system to confirm that the amount of the approved adjustment matches the adjustment actually posted.

3. For narrative purposes, note any significant processing delays.

4. If the audit identifies a processing error, identify the specific error and include the error information in the audit report and work papers.

5. Detailed work papers should be prepared and provided as backup to the audit report.

Figure 4.11 — Sample approved charity application audit worksheet

Acct #	DOS	Complete application (Y/N)	Eligibility correct (Y/N)	W/O per form ($)	W/O per system ($)	Variance ($)	Audit issue (Y/N)
245628-7	12/5/04	Y	Y	$750.00	$650.00	$10.00	Y—late credit

Note: This worksheet is included on the accompanying CD-ROM.

The summary of this data includes the following:

- Percentage of complete applications
- Percentage of applications correctly classified as eligible
- Percentage of adjustment variances
- Average adjustment variance dollar value

The audit report typically includes a methodology statement that describes how you selected the sample and the size of the sample. Document all the tasks performed in the audit. Also present a summary data table and highlight significant issues in a narrative section. Finally, include the auditor's recommendations for process improvement in the document. Provide the completed set of work papers with appropriate removal of protected health information (PHI).

Denied charity applications audit

To audit denied charity applications, select a random sample of 50–100 accounts processed within the most recent quarter. Alternatively, select a random sample equal to 20%–25% of all denied charity applications for the most recent quarter. If you need a statistical basis, use the sample size calculator found at *www.surveysystem.com/sscalc.htm*.

Using a worksheet, capture the following data for each account:

1. Review the eligibility determination against the charity policy and procedures and income guidelines in effect as of the determination date.

2. Trace the denial to the detailed patient account in the system to confirm that staff noted the denial and appropriately communicated it to the patient.

3. Confirm that staff sent patient statements following the charity denial.

4. For narrative purposes, note any significant processing delays.

5. If the audit identifies a processing error, identify the specific error and include the error information in the audit report and work papers.

6. Detailed work papers should be prepared and provided as backup to the audit report.

Figure	4.12	Sample denied charity application audit worksheet

Acct #	DOS	Account balance	Status: A/R or bad debt	Payment plan (Y/N)	PP months to resolve	Denial correct (Y/N)	Denial reason (code)
165803-7	11/15/04	$24592.18	A/R	Y	246	N	4

Note: This worksheet is included on the accompanying CD-ROM.

The summary of this data includes the following:

- Percentage of correct denials
- Percentage of denied applications in A/R
- Percentage of denied applications in bad debt
- Percentage of denied accounts with payment plans
- Average number of months to resolve payment plans
- Denial percentages by denial codes

The audit report typically includes a methodology statement that describes how you selected the sample and the size of the sample. Document all the tasks performed in the audit. Also present a summary data table and highlight significant issues in a narrative section. Finally, include the auditor's recommendations for process improvement in the document. Provide the completed set of work papers with appropriate removal of PHI.

Payment plan audit

Use an audit of payment plan accounts to identify accounts that staff may have overlooked for charity processing. To select a random sample, obtain a system-generated report listing all payment plans for dates of service within the most recent six-month period. Determine the sample size based on the number of payment plans, the confidence interval, and confidence level needed. You can use the sample calculator found at *www.surveysystem.com/sscalc.htm* to find the sample size.

Once you have selected the random sample, individually review the accounts in the patient accounting system. Before starting the review, obtain a copy of the hospital's current payment plan account, as well as any older versions of the policy that may have been in effect during the audit period. The sample worksheet in Figure 4.13 has been successfully used in payment plan auditing:

| Figure | 4.13 | Sample payment plan audit |

Acct # or ref. #	Current balance due	Required pay plan amount per month per policy	Negotiated amount accepted	# Missing or late payments	# Months to resolve at current rate	Resolution beyond payment plan policy (Y/N)	Review for charity (Y/N)
125	$4,600	$150	$100	2	46	Y	Y

Note: This worksheet is included on the accompanying CD-ROM.

Because the purpose of this audit is to identify possible charity accounts, an important calculation revolves around the duration of the payment plan. Any account that will not be resolved within the time frame permitted in the payment plan policy should be reviewed for possible charity consideration, as well as sale or outsourcing, as appropriate.

This data includes

- average payment plan balance
- average variance between required payment and negotiated payment
- average number of missing or late payments
- average number of months to resolve
- number of accounts out of compliance with payment plan policy
- number of accounts selected for further charity review

The audit report typically includes a methodology statement that describes how you selected the sample and the size of the sample. Document all of the tasks performed in the audit. Also present a summary data table and highlight significant issues in a narrative section. Finally, include the auditor's recommendations for process improvement in the document. Provide the completed set of work papers with appropriate removal of PHI.

Summary

There are a number of assessment techniques that you may use to determine the state of charity processing within your organization. Each assessment provides a different view of the current process. By combining several assessments, PFS directors and their staff can develop an accurate profile of the opportunities and magnitude of the changes that could be implemented to improve efficiency and increase patient satisfaction. Finally, the risk assessment becomes an educational tool for the project team responsible for developing and implementing revisions to the current charity processes.

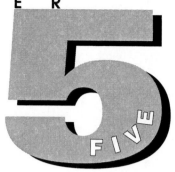
Best practices: The ideal revenue cycle and charity processing

Best practices: The ideal revenue cycle and charity processing

The ideal revenue cycle process recognizes that the provision of care is an extension of both clinical and financial care. The revenue cycle begins when the physician and patient identify a need for a clinical service. For some patients, the cycle begins in the physician's office when the physician writes the order for a test or treatment, including surgery, and schedules the work with the hospital. For other patients, the cycle begins in the hospital's emergency department (ED) when the patient arrives for an unscheduled urgent or emergent service. Still other patients come to the hospital for services that are routinely scheduled (e.g., routine laboratory services).

This book differentiates the best practices and the ideal revenue cycle and charity workflows based on the scheduled or unscheduled nature of the encounter, instead of differentiating between inpatient and outpatient status. This approach standardizes processing requirements for all encounters. However, the significant variable is when the provider becomes aware of the patient's intent to receive a service. In other words, the provider becomes aware of the service request at the time of scheduling for scheduled patients. However, emergency and walk-in patients come to the provider's attention when they arrive and request a service.

As a result of increased processing activity during the pre-service and time of service phases of the revenue cycle, the timing of processing is shifting into these phases. An excellent example of this shift is charity processing. Providers are viewing charity processing as more than just a post-service, collections department activity. In a recent HCPro survey, charity processing has moved into the earlier parts of the revenue cycle process, confirming that addressing patient financial concerns at an early opportunity is a patient-friendly approach.

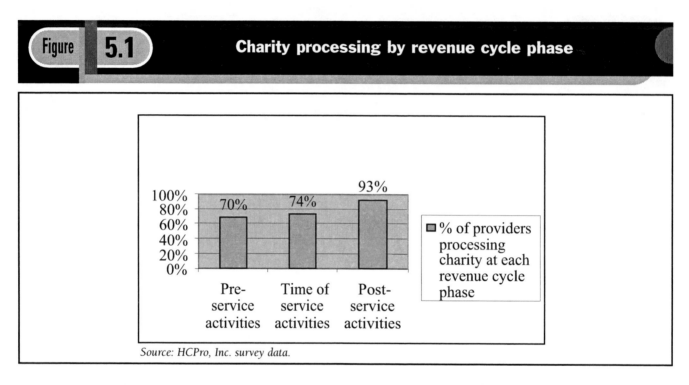

Figure 5.1   **Charity processing by revenue cycle phase**

Source: HCPro, Inc. survey data.

Pre-service processing: Scheduled patient workflow

Pre-service revenue cycle activities include all functions that ensure comprehensive patient financial and customer service processing before providing scheduled services.

1. Reservation for service

The patient or the physician's office initiates the reservation for service, and the hospital obtains the electronic comprehensive data set at that time. Alternatively, the patient provides the required data set either via the telephone or, preferably, via the Internet. Internet access includes a secure data transfer approach. The patient completes a form, the form is system-checked for completion of required fields, and then the form is transmitted to the provider for processing. This allows the hospital staff to identify the patient within the hospital database, confirm that either the physician or the patient has obtained all managed care authorizations, and initiate the verification of insurance coverage. If the database does not identify the patient, the reservation data set transaction initiates a new master patient record and automatically notifies hospital personnel that new patient processing is required.

2. Scheduling initiated

While the hospital creates or updates the enterprise master patient index, the resource scheduling processor identifies the place, service, equipment, personnel resource(s), and date and time available for the service requested. The system records the tentative scheduling transaction and issues an electronic notification to the appropriate clinical and business personnel.

3. Clinical requirements resolved

Clinical prerequisites (e.g., pre-service testing, medical necessity compliance requirements, medical records requests, patient assessment, etc.) are system-identified based on a comprehensive service requirements matrix. To make this happen, the pre-admission nurse confirms the requirements and contacts the patient to discuss the pre-service testing requirements and to complete the patient assessment. During this call, the nurse tells the patient to expect a follow-up call from patient financial services (PFS) personnel to review insurance eligibility and benefits, any outstanding managed care issues, and financial assistance, as appropriate. The pre-admission nurse or other clinician completes the medical necessity screening to ensure that the proposed services, diagnostic information, physician orders, and other clinical factors are sufficiently documented as required by payer regulations or contract terms. When pre-service testing is complete, the nurse reviews the results and contacts the physician to discuss any problems or concerns identified through the testing and assessment process.

Medical necessity screening is completed based on Medicare and other payer requirements. The physician's order, including diagnostic information, is used to complete the screening process. If the requested service fails to meet medical necessity standards, the physician is contacted to attempt to resolve the issue. If the service is truly medically unnecessary and, therefore, not covered by the patient's insurance plan, that information is shared with the patient during the financial education contact.

4. Insurance processing

After the hospital has created or updated the master patient record, PFS staff electronically complete the insurance verification to confirm eligibility and benefits, including the details of the benefit package. The hospital captures and stores benefit information electronically, including inpatient benefits for all levels of service, home health benefits, and outpatient benefits, including restrictions such as laboratory contracts. *Note:* In today's self-insured environment, the employer often maintains eligibility files and the plan's third-party administrator often houses benefit files.

For Medicare patients, the hospital completes Medicare secondary payer screening and uses the information to establish the appropriate sequencing of the patient's Medicare plan and other insurance plans. For example, if the patient or the patient's spouse is employed, has coverage for the patient through an employer group health plan, and has an employer with at least 20 employees, then the group health plan becomes the primary insurance. Medicare is sequenced as the secondary payer. Other Medicare secondary payer screening issues include black lung coverage, veterans administration coverage, worker's compensation, disability, end-stage renal disease, and liability situations. Check your screening form requirements to determine whether any of these situations apply.

The hospital checks managed care contracts against the insurance information and obtains any required certification during the reservation contact. PFS staff then assign approval information to single or multiple visits, as needed. Authorization information is electronically passed to case management personnel for use during inpatient recertification reviews.

5. Charge anticipation

After the hospital verifies insurance, PFS staff anticipate charges based on the clinical information originally provided by the patient or physician. The hospital then contacts the patient. A primary objective of this communication is to inform the patient of the organization's financial policies and the activities that will take place throughout the continuum of the patient's care. As appropriate, PFS staff initiate screening for charity eligibility at this time.

6. Completion of patient pre-service processing

PFS staff provide patients with specific financial education to confirm the results of the insurance verification contact, discuss the specific patient liability and resolution, and explain other issues that require the patient's involvement, such as the presentation of claim forms. Once staff have resolved these issues, the patient is qualified for a courtesy admission. The patient is directed to proceed directly to the service area on the day of service. Hospital staff change the tentative reservation to a confirmed reservation and the physician, service department(s), and patient electronically receive a pre-service notification to confirm the date and time of the scheduled service. Staff may also provide the confirmation via fax or telephone.

7. Patient arrival—Date of service

On the scheduled date of service, face sheets, consent forms, and Health Insurance Portability and Accountability Act of 1996 (HIPAA) privacy notification forms, as needed, are delivered by admissions staff to each point-of-service location or, ideally, routed to high-speed printers in each point-of-service area. Alternatively, staff route the forms to printers in a central patient access location and sort the forms appropriately. Because staff have previously validated the patient's demographic and financial information, the arrival process is expedited. Patient signatures and any required payments are obtained by either the service area staff or admissions staff, and the patient receives the scheduled service(s).

Summary

In this model, the patient is appropriately educated and the hospital resolves all financial processing issues before the patient receives the service. This results in higher patient satisfaction levels, improved collections, and reduced levels of bad debt because the patient has negotiated and agreed to the financial outcome before receiving the service. The hospital also identifies and resolves charity eligibility, thus reducing post-service collection efforts and costs. Further, the clinical pre-service processing ensures that medical necessity and pre-service testing requirements are met before the date of service, which reduces the chance of a last-minute cancellation.

Pre-service charity processing details

Opportunities to initiate the charity application and approval process exist within the pre-service workflow. For the individual hospital, these opportunities occur after staff have completed the insurance verification process and before the patient arrives for service. Specifically, once the staff complete the insurance verification, the provider has determined not only whether the patient is eligible for insurance coverage, but also the details of that benefit package. The hospital can typically base processing activities thereafter on the type of payer.

For contracted and government payers, PFS staff anticipate the charges for the proposed service and apply the contract or governmental payer payment structure as appropriate. For some government programs, such as Medicaid, unless the patient has a spend-down liability (i.e., the amount the patient must pay for medical care before Medicaid becomes effective), the payment the hospital receives will be payment in full. Medicare, however, has deductible and coinsurance requirements that result in balances after the application of the Medicare payment. Therefore, hospitals anticipate a secondary insurance or patient liability for these patients. For managed care plans, patients may owe a deductible and a coinsurance amount. Understanding exactly how each contracted payer adjudicates the benefit package provided to the patient is vital to accurate calculations. Once the hospital has completed the insurance processing, staff contact the patient and provide financial education. During this conversation, the hospital has the opportunity to discuss the results of the verification activity, to discuss any identified patient liability, and to identify the most appropriate account resolution option through dialog with the patient.

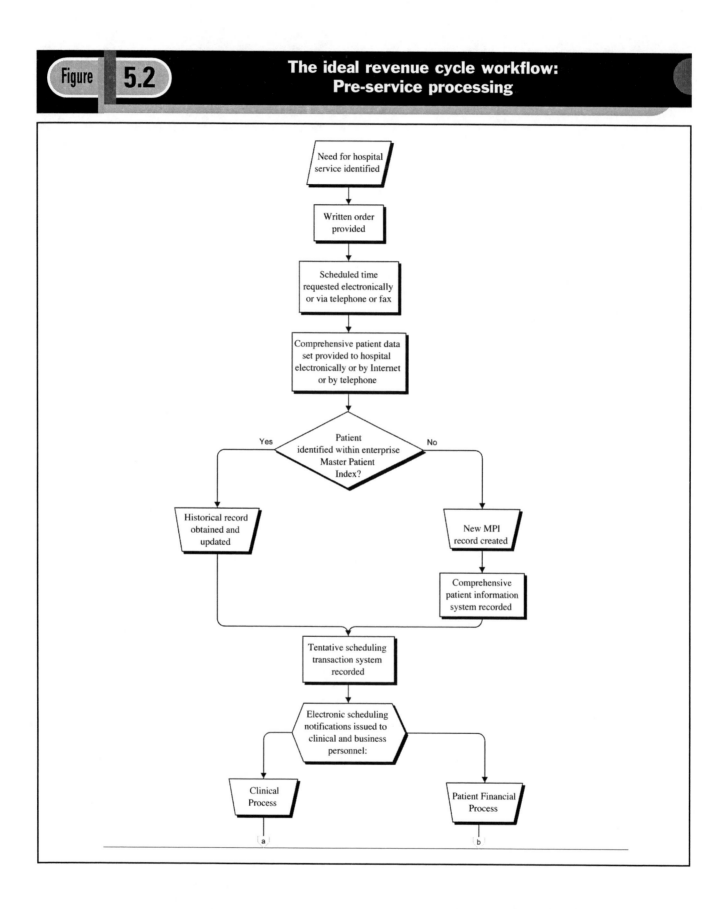

Figure 5.2

**The ideal revenue cycle workflow:
Pre-service processing**

Need for hospital
service identified

Written order
provided

Scheduled time
requested electronically
or via telephone or fax

Comprehensive patient data
set provided to hospital
electronically or by Internet
or by telephone

Patient
identified within enterprise
Master Patient
Index?

Yes — Historical record
obtained and
updated

No — New MPI
record created

Comprehensive
patient information
system recorded

Tentative scheduling
transaction system
recorded

Electronic scheduling
notifications issued to
clinical and business
personnel:

Clinical
Process

Patient Financial
Process

a

b

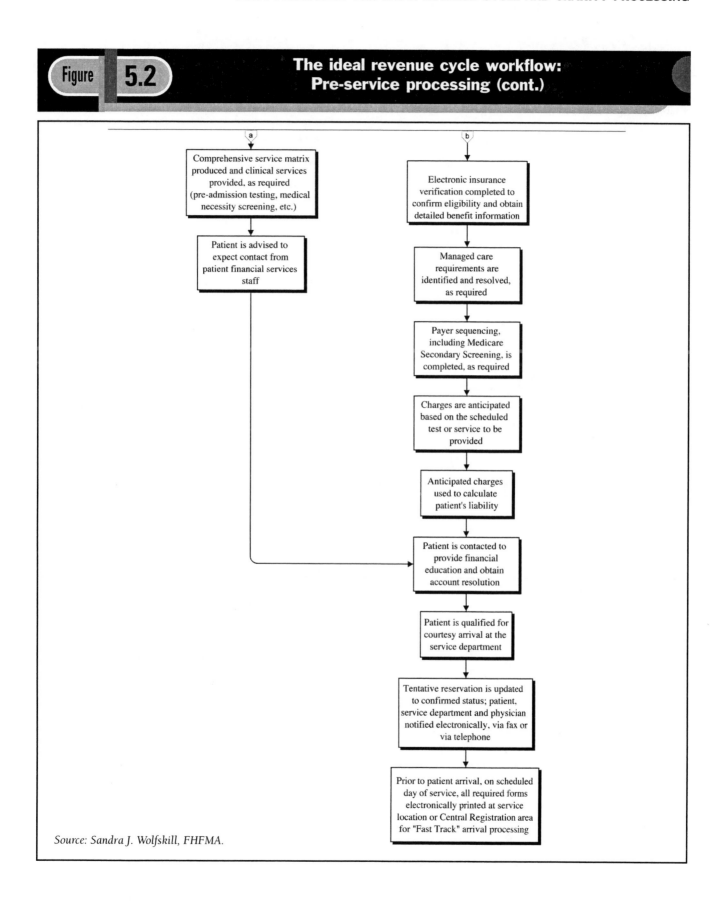

Figure 5.2

**The ideal revenue cycle workflow:
Pre-service processing (cont.)**

a

Comprehensive service matrix produced and clinical services provided, as required (pre-admission testing, medical necessity screening, etc.)

Patient is advised to expect contact from patient financial services staff

b

Electronic insurance verification completed to confirm eligibility and obtain detailed benefit information

Managed care requirements are identified and resolved, as required

Payer sequencing, including Medicare Secondary Screening, is completed, as required

Charges are anticipated based on the scheduled test or service to be provided

Anticipated charges used to calculate patient's liability

Patient is contacted to provide financial education and obtain account resolution

Patient is qualified for courtesy arrival at the service department

Tentative reservation is updated to confirmed status; patient, service department and physician notified electronically, via fax or via telephone

Prior to patient arrival, on scheduled day of service, all required forms electronically printed at service location or Central Registration area for "Fast Track" arrival processing

Source: Sandra J. Wolfskill, FHFMA.

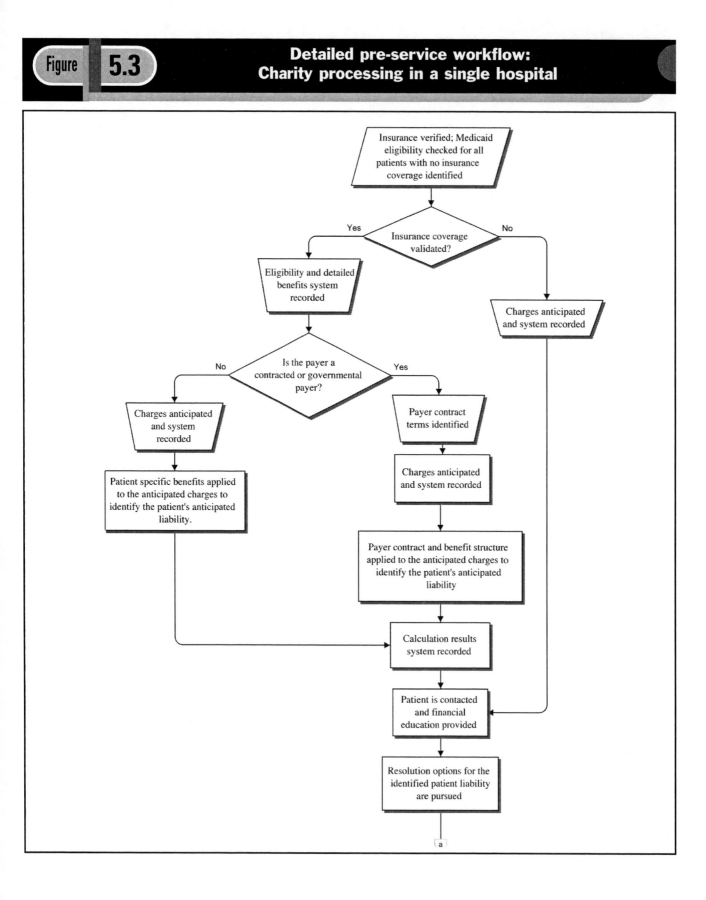

Figure 5.3

**Detailed pre-service workflow:
Charity processing in a single hospital**

Figure 5.3 — Detailed pre-service workflow: Charity processing in a single hospital (cont.)

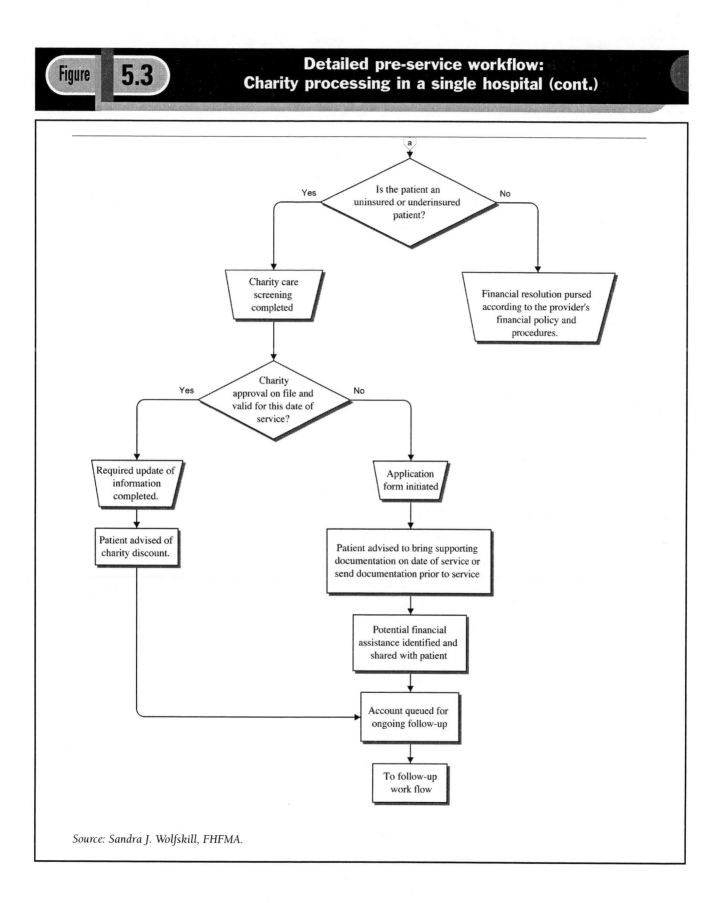

Source: *Sandra J. Wolfskill, FHFMA.*

For non-government, non-contracted payers, there is no discounting provision in place between the payer and the provider. Therefore, the payer should adjudicate the claim based on the patient's benefit package. Understanding the benefits available allows provider staff to accurately calculate the anticipated patient liability.

If staff determine that the patient is uninsured or underinsured, staff identify and share the potential financial assistance with the patient. If the patient has a pre-existing charity application on file, staff review and confirm the applicability to the proposed service. If not, staff may initiate the new charity application and explain the documentation during a telephone call. Patients may have the option to mail the documentation or provide it in person on the day of service. Based on the preliminary information, staff can determine the amount of financial assistance and share this with the patient. Staff then route the account into a specific charity service follow-up queue so that it goes to the appropriate area for additional follow-up and processing. Staff identify and establish appropriate follow-up activities based on each subsequent conversation with the patient.

Integrated delivery system

The integrated delivery system provides different opportunities for charity processing. In a completely integrated model, whether in multiple facilities or in an integrated teaching hospital and faculty group, charity policies and procedures are standardized and applied uniformly across the enterprise. This results in higher patient satisfaction and reduced patient confusion because the enterprise is presenting a single approach and a single set of rules to the patient population.

In the integrated model, a central data repository contains the approved charity applications for all patients. Individual service providers have access to the centralized applications and make charity determinations based on the information gathered by the first provider to service the patient. Applications are valid for a pre-determined time frame, and all providers follow a common eligibility determination procedure. When a charity determination expires, the next provider to service the patient automatically initiates and completes a renewal application, which it then approves or rejects based on the patient's current financial situation.

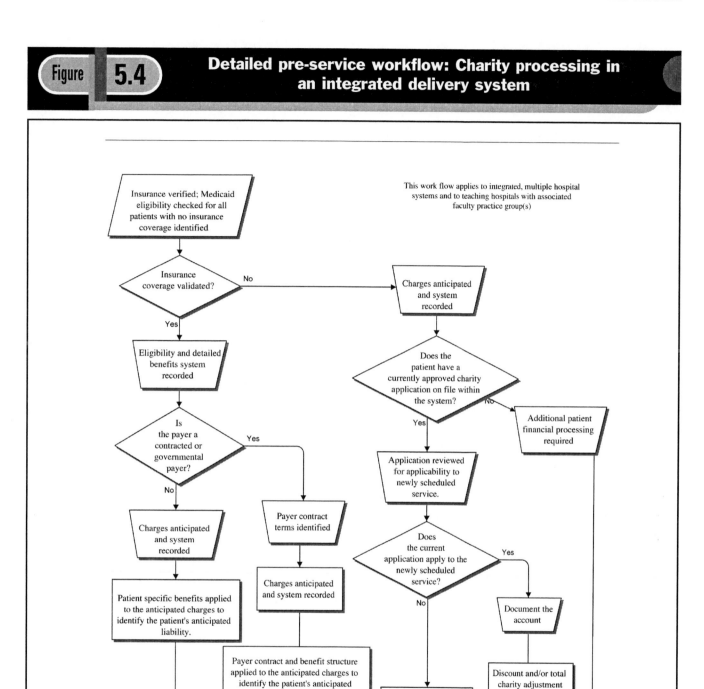

Figure 5.4 — Detailed pre-service workflow: Charity processing in an integrated delivery system

Insurance verified; Medicaid eligibility checked for all patients with no insurance coverage identified

This work flow applies to integrated, multiple hospital systems and to teaching hospitals with associated faculty practice group(s)

Insurance coverage validated? → No → Charges anticipated and system recorded

Yes

Eligibility and detailed benefits system recorded

Is the payer a contracted or governmental payer?

Yes → Payer contract terms identified

No

Charges anticipated and system recorded

Patient specific benefits applied to the anticipated charges to identify the patient's anticipated liability.

Charges anticipated and system recorded

Payer contract and benefit structure applied to the anticipated charges to identify the patient's anticipated liability

Calculation results system recorded

Patient is contacted and financial education provided

a

Does the patient have a currently approved charity application on file within the system?

Yes → Application reviewed for applicability to newly scheduled service.

No → Additional patient financial processing required

Does the current application apply to the newly scheduled service?

Yes → Document the account

No → Review documentation updated in system

Discount and/or total charity adjustment applied appropriately.

Patient contacted to provide financial education and pursue resolution of any residual patient liability.

Figure 5.4 Detailed pre-service workflow: Charity processing in an integrated delivery system (cont.)

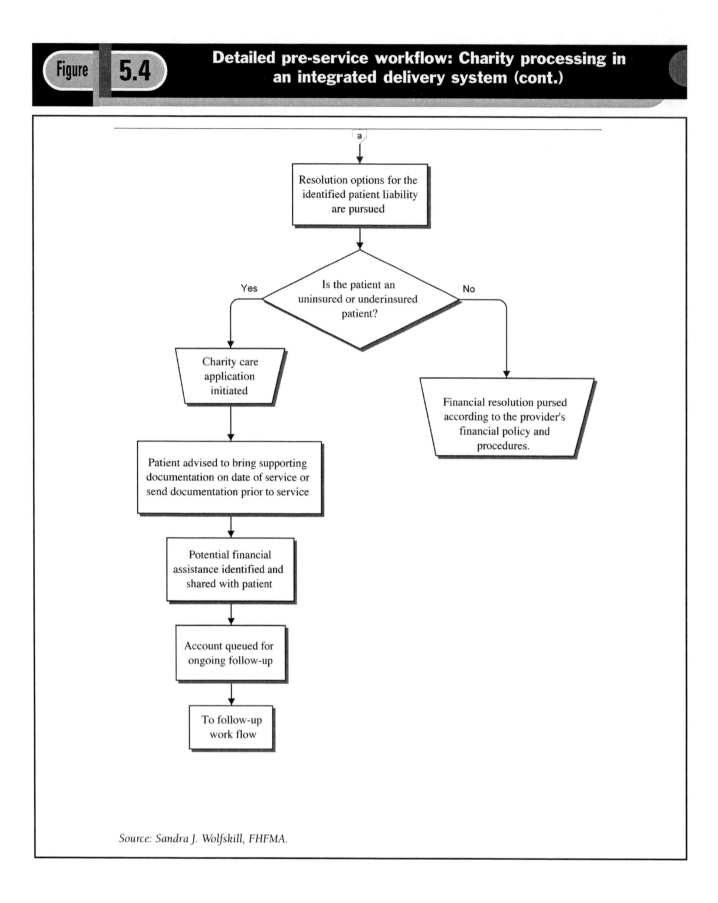

Source: Sandra J. Wolfskill, FHFMA.

Time of service processing: Scheduled patient workflow

Time of service processing includes two groups of patients: those scheduled and those not scheduled for service. For the scheduled patient, this phase of the revenue cycle involves patient arrival processing and provision of service.

1. Patient arrival

Time of service processing includes all activities that occur from the time the patient arrives for service through the patient's discharge or exit from the facility. Immediately before the patient's arrival, nursing personnel complete bed assignments for all scheduled inpatients. For all scheduled services, the patient reports to the information desk and is directed to the service area. Arrival processing is done in the service area because the patient completed the pre-service processing requirements, including pre-registration, insurance verification, patient financial education, etc., having received point of service access status during the pre-service process. State-of-the-art way-finding tools (e.g., directional signs) are employed to ensure easy access to all service units. Alternatively, the patient arrives at the central registration area, where pre-processed patients are expedited through a "fast track" or "express" access desk. Upon arrival at the service unit or central registration fast track/express area, staff activate the patient's registration record, document the arrival time, and complete any edits that remain unresolved from the pre-service process. The patient then is directed by the clinical clerk or admissions staff to the service area and services are provided.

2. Service-related activities

The additional activities during this period include ongoing medical necessity screening, order entry, results reporting, posting of charges, concurrent entry of diagnostic and procedural coding as results are made available to coding personnel, monitoring of charges and coverage levels v. the original projections, resolution of additional patient liabilities, monitoring and resolution of ongoing managed care requirements, completion of discharge planning screens, and completion of all bill edits. Thus, during the provision of service period, the hospital resolves all required financial counseling activities. The nursing units also routinely complete the ongoing census management for inpatients and observation patients. The final aspect of time of service processing is the courtesy discharge of the patient directly from the nursing unit or service area, allowing the patient to leave the facility without delay.

Time of service processing: Unscheduled patient workflow

For the unscheduled patient, time of service activities include all activities required to process a patient, including registration, insurance verification, managed care resolution, medical necessity screening, charge anticipation, financial education and resolution, and provision of clinical services.

1. Patient arrival

For unscheduled patients, processing begins as the patient arrives for a service. The registration department creates the record by collecting demographic and insurance information (the traditional registration process). However, for unscheduled patients, the hospital must immediately initiate and systematically complete all of the previously defined pre-service activities for the scheduled patient (e.g., insurance verification, managed care screening, financial counseling, medical necessity screening, and documentation). Because of high-volume, low-dollar value services often provided in the outpatient setting, many providers use a threshold concept to determine when financial counseling is required. However, as more electronic insurance verification options become available, providers will be able to verify all insurance coverage during the registration process and provide financial counseling as needed to resolve accounts.

2. Emergency department

The time of service workflow within the ED is typically different from other unscheduled patient processing within the revenue cycle. For ED patients, the initial task is to identify the patient in the master patient index and create a visit record. Triage occurs to ensure proper sequencing of patients into the treatment area. The ED provides the medical screening examination and provides necessary services. Once the patient is stable, the registration staff complete a comprehensive bedside registration. Additional processing includes insurance verification, managed care screening, medical necessity screening, and preparation for the financial discharge interview. Preparation includes anticipation of charges, identification of patient copayment or coinsurance amounts, and application of the benefit plan(s) to the total charges. A financial interview follows the ED's clinical discharge process. The financial counselor or registration staff provide patient financial education and account resolution. If the ED admits the patient, the financial processing occurs on the nursing unit at the earliest appropriate opportunity.

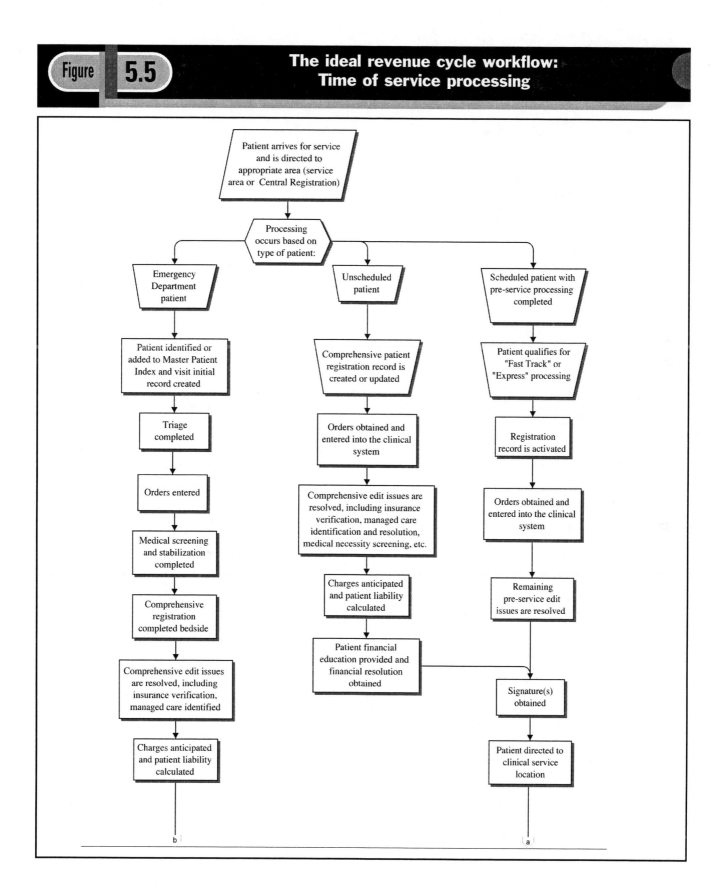

Figure 5.5

The ideal revenue cycle workflow: Time of service processing

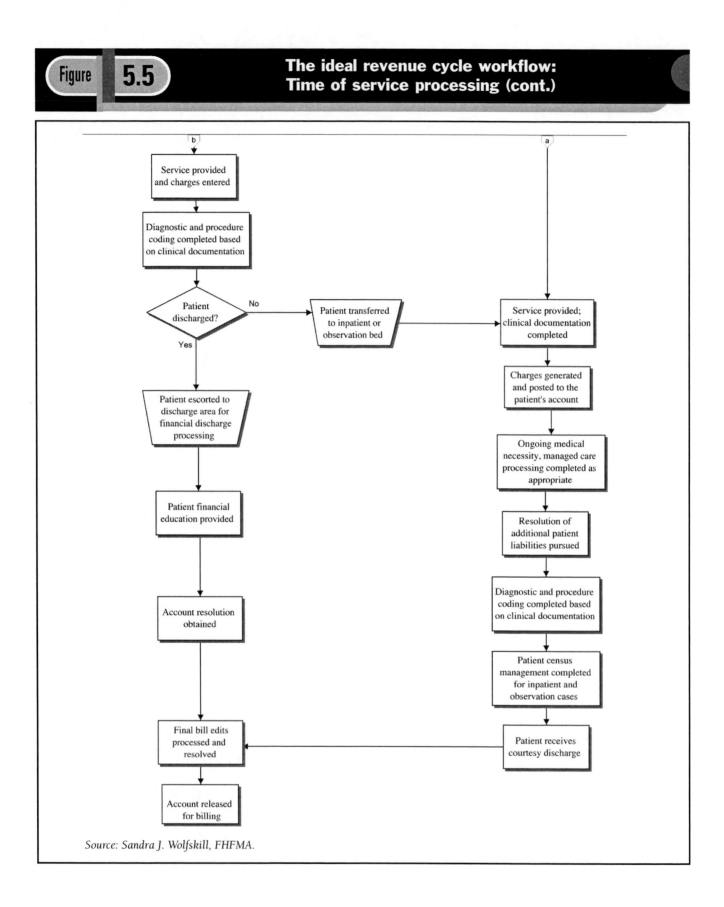

Figure 5.5

The ideal revenue cycle workflow: Time of service processing (cont.)

Source: Sandra J. Wolfskill, FHFMA.

Time of service charity processing details

Time of service charity processing details will vary depending on the scheduled or unscheduled nature of the service the hospital is providing. For scheduled patients, time of service activities typically focus on completing work initiated during the pre-service phase. For unscheduled patients, the charity process is more extensive because no processing has occurred prior to the patient's arrival for service.

1. Scheduled patient: Charity processing

At individual hospitals, opportunities to complete the charity application and approval process exist within the time of service workflow for the scheduled patient. Because the PFS staff financially educate and counsel scheduled patients prior to services, the patient access staff have system-generated alerts identifying the additional charity processing required when the patient arrives for service. Patient access staff print an application for the patient to sign, then scan and electronically insert attachments provided by the patient into the patient's electronic financial folder. Patient access staff then move the account into the final approval queue for priority review and processing by assigned personnel. Once approved, the system automatically posts the approved adjustment to ensure appropriate billing to the patient. Based on the approval result, the system produces and mails a system-generated notification to the patient. If a patient balance remains, the system automatically queues the account for appropriate follow-up based on the terms of the financial resolution conversation with the patient.

2. ED patient: Charity processing

Within the ED time of service process, while the patient receives treatment, PFS staff verify insurance, resolve managed care issues, and system record the patient's benefits. Specifically, once staff have completed insurance verification, the provider has determined not only whether the patient is eligible for insurance coverage, but also the details of that benefit package. Staff then typically base processing activities on the type of payer.

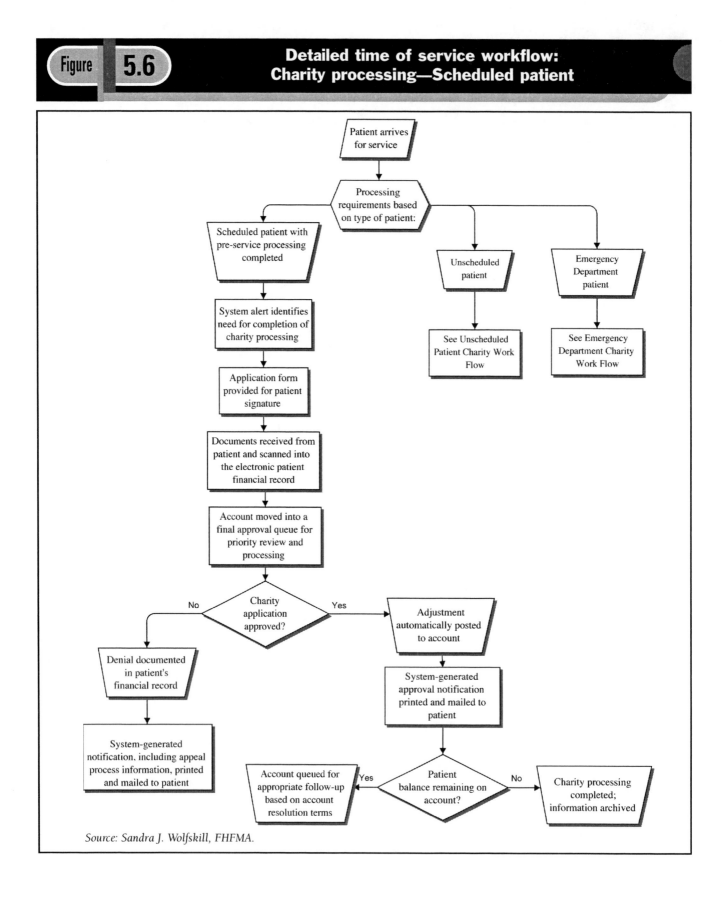

Figure 5.6 Detailed time of service workflow: Charity processing—Scheduled patient

Patient arrives for service

Processing requirements based on type of patient:

Scheduled patient with pre-service processing completed

System alert identifies need for completion of charity processing

Application form provided for patient signature

Documents received from patient and scanned into the electronic patient financial record

Account moved into a final approval queue for priority review and processing

Charity application approved?

No → Denial documented in patient's financial record → System-generated notification, including appeal process information, printed and mailed to patient

Yes → Adjustment automatically posted to account

System-generated approval notification printed and mailed to patient

Patient balance remaining on account?

Yes → Account queued for appropriate follow-up based on account resolution terms

No → Charity processing completed; information archived

Unscheduled patient → See Unscheduled Patient Charity Work Flow

Emergency Department patient → See Emergency Department Charity Work Flow

Source: Sandra J. Wolfskill, FHFMA.

For contracted and government payers, staff anticipate the charges for the ED service and apply the contract or governmental payer payment structure as appropriate. For some government programs, such as Medicaid, unless the patient has a spend-down liability, the payment received will be payment in full. Medicare, however, has deductible and coinsurance requirements that result in balances after the application of the Medicare payment. Therefore, for these patients, staff anticipate a secondary insurance or patient liability. For managed care plans, patients may owe a deductible or a coinsurance amount. Understanding exactly how each contracted payer adjudicates the benefit package provided to the patient is vital to accurate calculations. Once staff complete the insurance processing, staff record the results and use them during the discharge financial interview.

When the hospital clinically discharges the patient, staff escort the patient to the financial discharge area and provide financial education. During this conversation, the hospital has the opportunity to discuss the results of the verification activity and any identified patient liability, and identify the most appropriate account resolution option through a dialogue with the patient.

For non-government, non-contracted payers, there is no discounting provision in place between the payer and the provider. Therefore, the payer is expected to adjudicate the claim based on the patient's benefit package. Understanding the benefits available allows provider staff to calculate accurately the anticipated patient liability.

If staff determine that the patient is uninsured or underinsured, staff identify and share potential financial assistance with the patient. If the patient has a pre-existing charity application on file, staff review and confirm the applicability to the current service. If no application is on file, staff initiate the new charity application during the interview and explain documentation requirements to the patient. Staff then give the patient the option to mail the documentation or provide it in person within two business days. Based on the preliminary information, staff can determine the amount of financial assistance available and share this information with the patient. Staff then route the account into a specific charity service follow-up queue so that as the account moves through the processing cycle, it automatically routes to the appropriate area for additional follow-up and processing. Staff identify and establish appropriate follow-up activities based on each subsequent conversation with the patient.

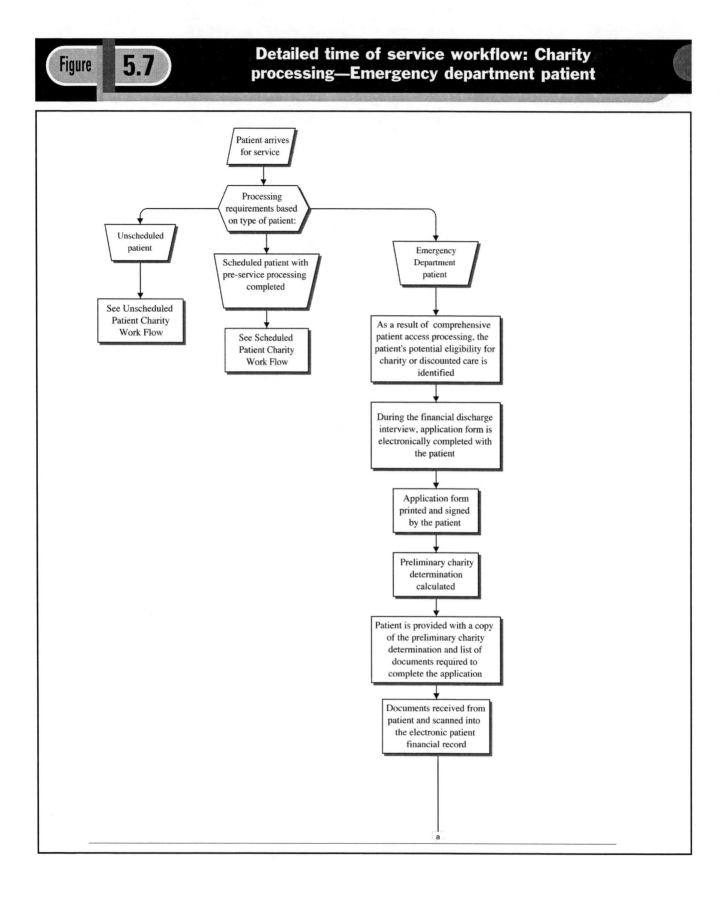

Figure 5.7 Detailed time of service workflow: Charity processing—Emergency department patient

Figure 5.7 | Detailed time of service workflow: Charity processing—Emergency department patient (cont.)

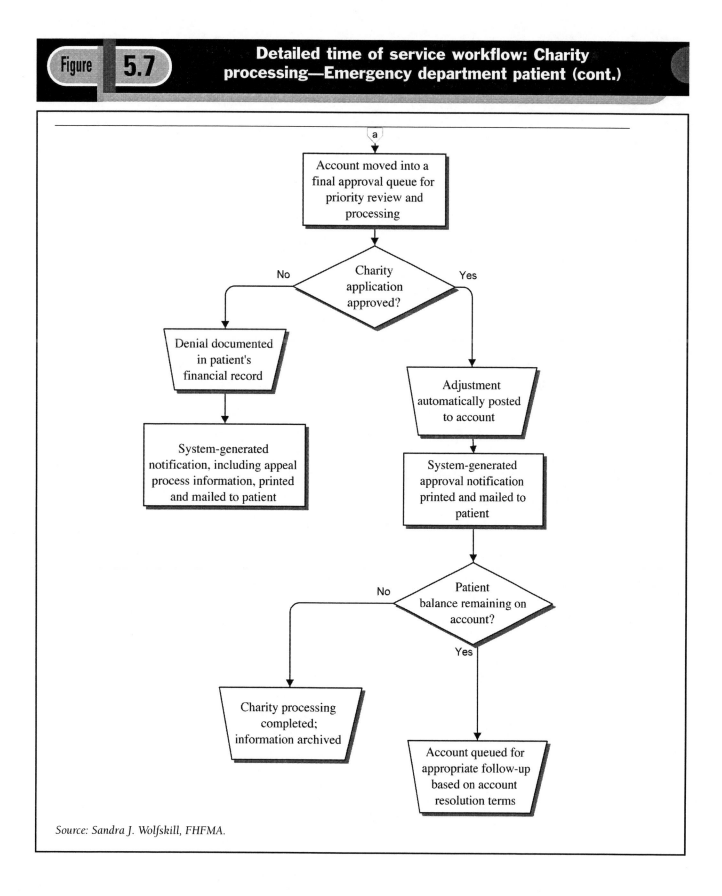

Source: Sandra J. Wolfskill, FHFMA.

3. Unscheduled patient: Charity processing

Staff should process all other unscheduled patients similarly. For these patients, however, the insurance verification, managed care resolution, medical necessity screening, charge anticipation, and benefit application occur during or immediately following the patient registration. Staff route patients with no identified liability directly to the service area, whereas staff route patients who qualify for financial counseling and potential charity screening to the financial counseling area for financial education.

If it is determined that the patient is uninsured or underinsured, potential financial assistance is identified and shared with the patient. If the patient has a pre-existing charity application on file, the applicability to the current service is reviewed and confirmed. If not, the new charity application is initiated during the interview and documentation requirements are explained to the patient. Patients are given the option to mail the documentation or provide it in person within two business days. Based on the preliminary information, the amount of financial assistance can be determined and shared with the patient. The account is then routed into a specific charity service follow-up queue so that as the account moves through the processing cycle, it is automatically routed to the appropriate area for additional follow-up and processing. Appropriate follow-up activities are identified and established based on each subsequent conversation with the patient.

4. Integrated delivery system: Charity processing

In the integrated delivery system model, the workflows are similar to the single hospital examples, except that the charity data is centrally stored and available to all providers within the integrated system.

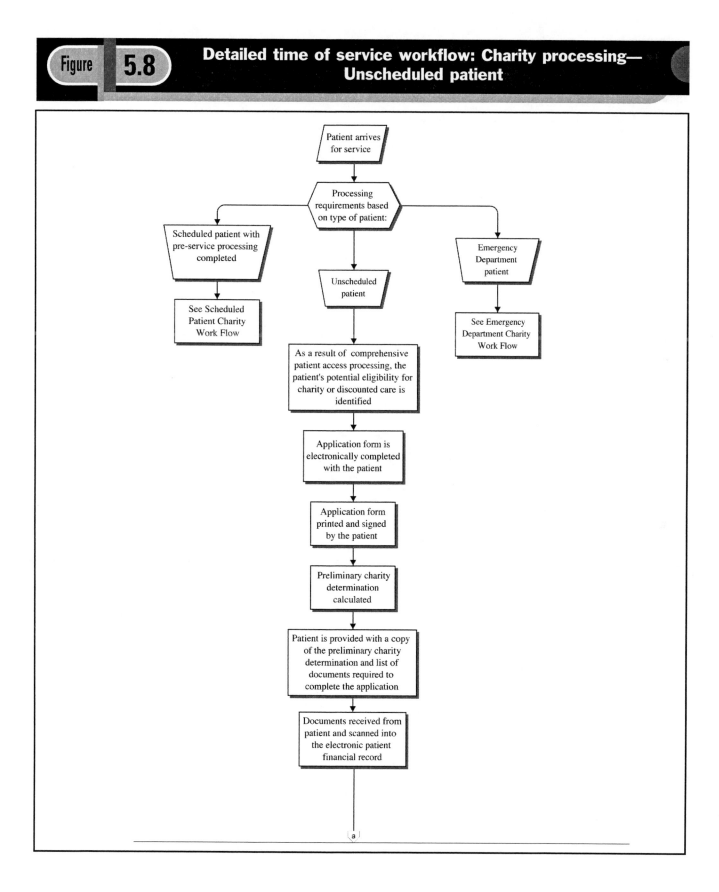

Figure 5.8 Detailed time of service workflow: Charity processing—Unscheduled patient

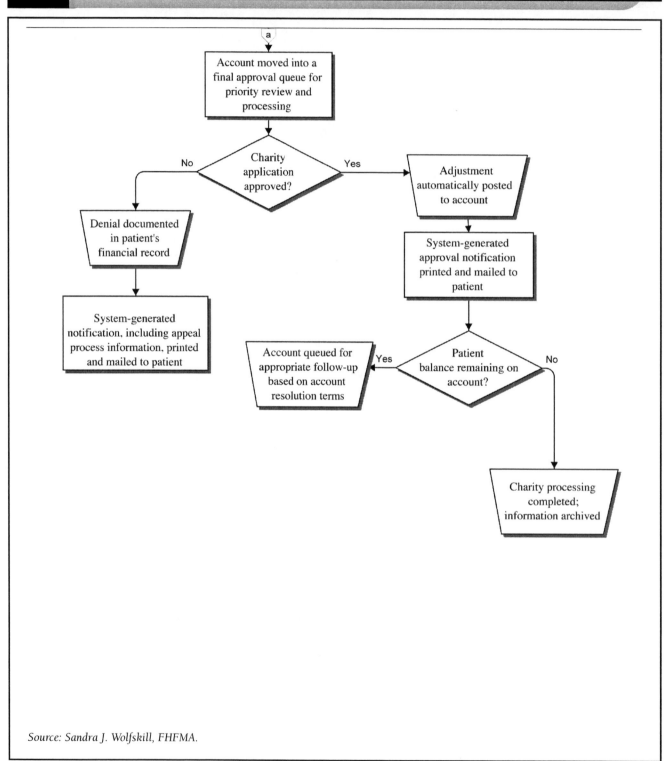

Source: Sandra J. Wolfskill, FHFMA.

Post-service processing

Regardless of the scheduled or unscheduled nature of a patient encounter, ultimately the facility provides the services and completes the treatment period. What remains are the activities needed to complete the financial processing of the patient's account.

Post-service processing includes all activities that the hospital must complete once the patient's treatment ends. This includes resolving the final billing edits and appropriately billing and resolving the account. The ideal pre-service and time of service flows result in the complete and accurate gathering of all information and the resolution of insurance verification, managed care issues, and charity/discount approval, as well as concurrent posting of charges and medical record coding. Therefore, after discharge, the facility holds the patient's account in a suspense or unbilled status for a minimal number of days. The number of suspense days should never exceed three days unless coding and charging issues cannot be resolved in that time frame. During this suspense period, a final compliance review ensures that the hospital does not submit fraudulent claims for payment. Electronic billing software performs the final compliance edits.

Post-service processing also includes the calculation and application of appropriate contractual adjustments based on the facility's contract with the identified primary payer. The hospital then produces and electronically submits an error-free, contractually adjusted claim for all bills, except those few bills that must be manually submitted to payers that are currently exempt from the HIPAA transaction set requirements. However, the hospital processes all claims through the comprehensive final edit system to ensure completion of all billing requirements. Staff identify and appropriately handle those claims requiring various attachments (e.g., medical records, claim forms, etc.) before billing. Staff automatically release lean claims (i.e., those claims with no electronic edit failures) daily to the indicated payers. Therefore, upon receipt of the Aclean electronic or paper claim, the payer is able to quickly process the bill for payment.

Upon release of the claim to the payer, the account is automatically queued into a rules-based account tracking system that monitors the account for payments and adjustments and appropriately assigns the account for processing according to the next required activity. Rules-based systems automate the account monitoring process and queue accounts for additional action as needed. If the accounts do not receive timely payments, the software immediately identifies the accounts for follow-up processing according to a defined time frame based on each payer's known Aclean claim cycle. In addition, because the financial counseling process identifies and resolves patient liabilities, no additional self-pay follow-up is required at this time and the system sends the patients or guarantors routine statements as appropriate, simultaneous with the initial third-party billing.

All contractual adjustments are accurately posted prior to billing, and charges are properly pro-rated. The hospital receives payments and posts them electronically. Simultaneously, the system applies billing and payment data to the appropriate payer log. As the system posts payments, accounts not fully resolved are identified as exceptions, analyzed, and appropriate action initiated (e.g., appeals to payers for under payments, initiation of secondary billing, etc.) by PFS staff. Because the hospital bills patient liabilities concurrently with insurance claims, the self-pay processing is reduced to automatic monitoring activity, with delinquent accounts system identified, and automatically transferred to a collection agency at predetermined intervals.

Once all charges are appropriately paid, the zero balance account is immediately archived by the system. Staff use appropriate storage and retrieval systems to retrieve the account should additional processing be required at a later time.

Post-service charity processing details

Historically, charity processing has occurred as a post-service activity. Once the patient received a bill for the patient portion, collection efforts would begin. During this process, the patient may indicate an inability to pay and, therefore, begin a discussion about charity or discounted care options.

Although in the ideal work environment charity activities would be completed prior to or no later than the patient's discharge, some charity processing may fall into the post-service phase of the revenue cycle. This may occur for several reasons:

1. Occasionally, a patient may fail to initiate a charity or discount application during the pre-service or time of service interviews. If staff later determine that the patient is uninsured or underinsured, the staff identifies and shares potential financial assistance with the patient.

2. If the patient has a pre-existing charity application on file, staff review and confirm the applicability to the current service. If no application is on file, staff initiate the new charity application and explain the documentation requirements to the patient. Staff then give patients the option to mail the documentation or provide it in person within two business days.

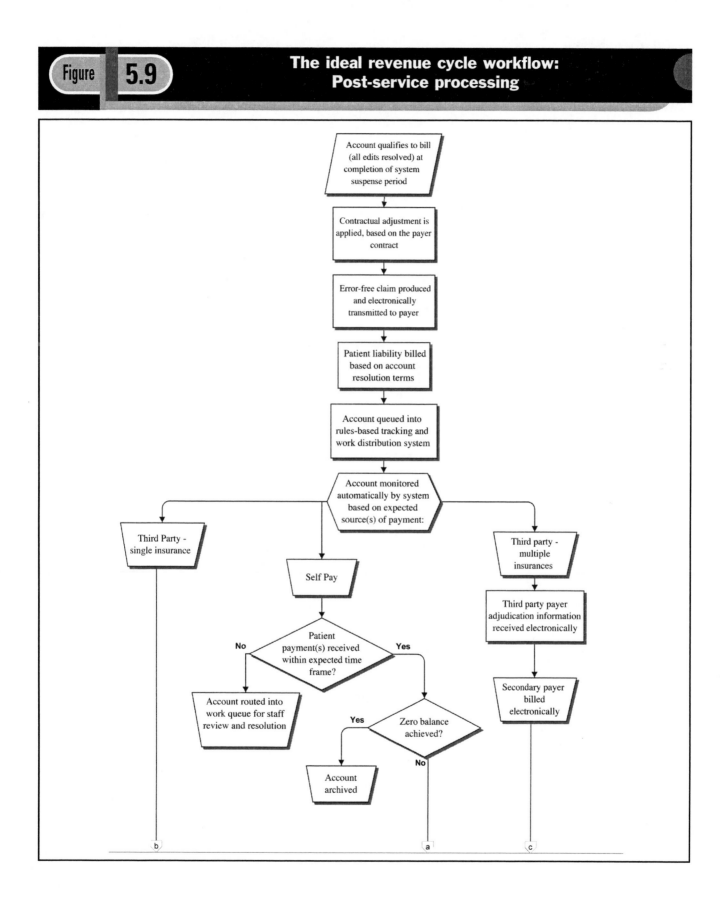

Figure 5.9

The ideal revenue cycle workflow: Post-service processing

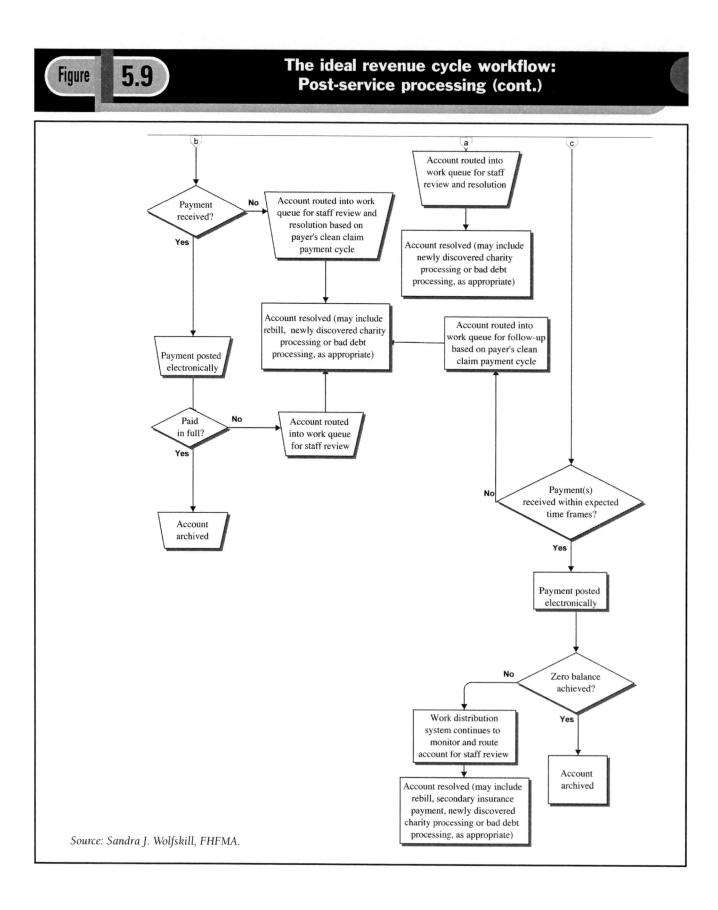

Figure 5.9 The ideal revenue cycle workflow: Post-service processing (cont.)

Source: Sandra J. Wolfskill, FHFMA.

3. Based on the preliminary information, staff can determine the amount of financial assistance and share this information with the patient. Staff then route the account into a specific charity service queue for additional follow-up and processing. Appropriate follow-up activities are system-identified based on the provider's established timeline for charity processing activities.

4. Multiple patient contacts may be completed in order to successfully assist the patient with the application process. Ultimately, the application is either completed and approved or it is denied and a system-generated notice is mailed to the patient. *Note:* The patient should be able to appeal a denied application through a formalized appeal process. The details of the appeal process should be included in the denial notice.

5. In the integrated delivery system model, the workflows are similar to the single hospital examples, except the charity data is centrally stored and available to all providers within the integrated system.

The charity application denial appeal process

Regardless of when the charity application is received by the hospital, the patient may disagree with the hospital's charity determination and appeal it. Therefore, a formal appeal process is an essential part of the overall charity process. During the appeal, the patient should be given the opportunity to present additional information relevant to the application. A different manager within the PFS area should be involved in reviewing and resolving the appeal. Ideally, a second level appeal to the chief financial officer ensures that patient concerns will receive a fair and timely hearing.

Figure 5.10 Detailed post-service work flow: Charity processing

Figure 5.10 Detailed post-service workflow: Charity processing (cont.)

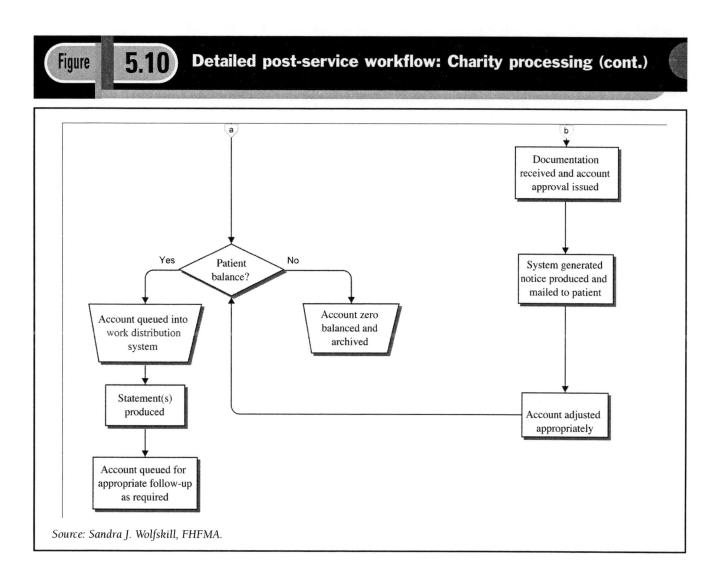

Source: Sandra J. Wolfskill, FHFMA.

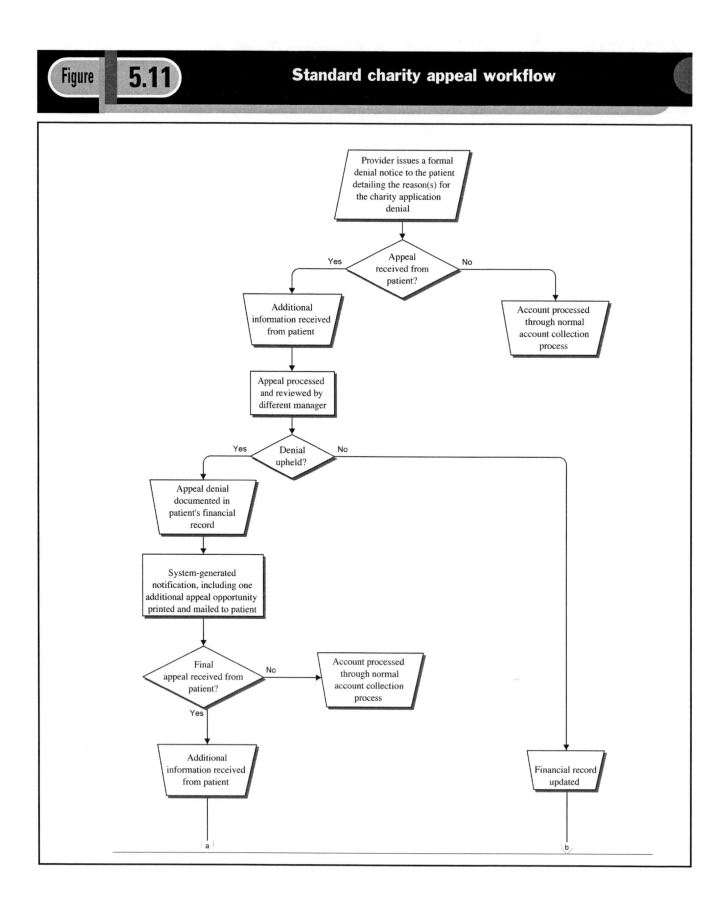

Figure 5.11 — Standard charity appeal workflow

Figure 5.11 — Standard charity appeal workflow (cont.)

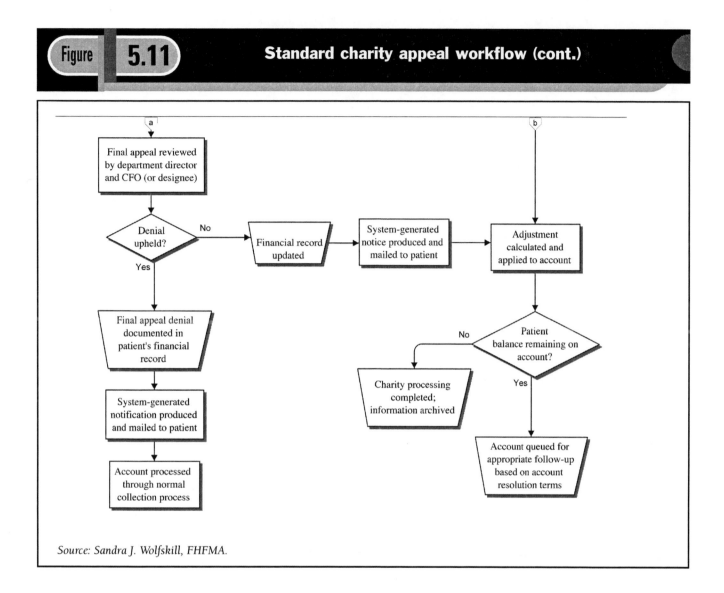

Source: Sandra J. Wolfskill, FHFMA.

Charity policies and procedures

Workflows are important tools for developing detailed policies and procedures. It is essential that throughout the revenue cycle we provide staff with documentation of the detailed activities required to complete charity processing. Because the required activities, the timing of activities, and the specific staff responsible for them will vary throughout the revenue cycle, care must be taken to customize policies—and especially procedures—to individual work environments.

| Figure | 5.12 | Detailed charity policy and procedures—Prototype document |

The following prototype charity and discount care policy follows the general outline of the workflows discussed in this chapter. Providers should add additional procedures to provide more specific, system-based activity definitions for all staff. Providers should also add suggested time frames for completion of the various activities based on the provider's overall revenue cycle process.

Subject: Charity and discounted care

Application: All departments

Purpose: To provide a reasonable amount of free or discounted care (i.e., uncompensated care) to patients who are unable to pay.

Policy: Recognizing its charitable mission, it is the policy of the hospital to provide a reasonable amount of its services without charge to eligible patients who cannot afford to pay for care. Discounted care will be provided to uninsured or underinsured patients who meet the established eligibility criteria and complete the required application and review process.

All medically necessary services of this facility will be available as uncompensated services.

Charity is defined as the demonstrated inability of a patient to pay. Bad debts are defined as the unwillingness of the patient to pay. Charity care does not include bad debt, contractual adjustments, or unreimbursed costs from other community services. The financial status of each patient should be determined so that an appropriate classification and distinction can be made between charity and bad debt. If the patient is able but unwilling to pay, the hospital will classify the account as bad debt.

Charity and discounted care include services provided to the following:

- Uninsured or underinsured low-income patients who do not have the ability to pay all or part of their bill as determined by the financial guidelines in this policy

- Insured patients whose coverage is inadequate to cover a catastrophic situation

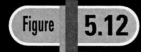

Detailed charity policy and procedures—Prototype document (cont.)

- Emergency patients, because the hospital does not assess a patient's financial situation before rendering services

- Persons whose income is sufficient to pay for basic living costs but not medical care, and also those persons with generally adequate incomes who are suddenly faced with catastrophically large medical bills

- Patients deemed medically indigent by virtue of their documented eligibility for Medicare and Medicaid benefits

A charity and discounted care budget will be established once a year during the annual budget process and submitted to the board of directors for approval. However, need for financial assistance will take priority over a fixed budget amount; the board will be promptly advised if charity and discounted care needs exceed the current budgetary provisions.

A formal appeal process shall be implemented to permit rapid review of all appealed charity denials. A charity committee shall be developed to review all final appeals of charity determinations.

Procedure:

1. Consider the following factors when determining the amount of charity service for which a patient is eligible at the time of service:

   - The patient should reside in the United States.

   - The patient's individual or family income, as appropriate, using the income guidelines in this policy, which take into consideration the cost of living for the community.

   - Individual or family net worth, including all liquid and convertible assets owned, less liabilities and claims against assets. The value of the patient's primary residence is excluded from the net worth calculation.

   - Employment status along with current earnings sufficient to meet the obligation within a

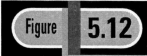

reasonable period of time. No more than "XX%" of the family income shall be considered available for purposes of a payment plan calculation; payment plan terms shall not be extended beyond the provider's normal payment plan program.

- Family size.

- Other financial obligations, including living expenses and other items of a reasonable and necessary nature.

- The amount(s) and frequency of hospital and other healthcare/medication bill(s) in relation to all of the factors outlined above. A patient may be deemed medically indigent when the only resources available for healthcare payment are Medicare and Medicaid benefits; for these patients, documentation should be developed. However, no additional collection efforts are required and the uncompensated amounts qualify for inclusion in the Medicare bad debt log.

- Medical indigence may also be determined for other patients. If the total outstanding medical bills for the patient exceed "$X" or "XX% of total assets," the medical indigent classification will apply and the patient will receive charity care.

- All other resources must be applied first, including third-party payers, Victims of Crime (i.e., a state-level program for crime victims to recover some hospital costs), and Medicaid. If a patient does not have Medicaid but would qualify, he or she must cooperate with the application process. If the application is denied or is identified as ineligible based on the Medicaid income criteria, consider for charity and discounted care.

2. Determine the appropriate amount of charity service in relation to the amounts due after applying all other resources. A patient who can afford to pay for a portion of the services will be expected to do so. *Note:* A third party might pay part of an account, the patient may pay part, and another part might meet charity services. If the patient does not pay the amount deemed to be his or her responsibility, the uncollectible remainder would become bad debt.

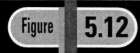

Detailed charity policy and procedures—Prototype document (cont.)

3. Require evidence of eligibility. Documentation should be submitted within "X" days of the date of service. Additional time for completion of the application process may be extended as needed. The patient must provide supporting documentation of income, which can include the following:

- Paycheck, general relief (i.e., a county-level public assistance program), Social Security, pension, unemployment or disability check stubs, tax return, or other proof of income.

- Application verification may include accessing the patient/guarantor's credit report. The patient must sign the charity form before accessing his or her credit information.

4. Send a letter to the attending physician to request that he or she extend charity to the patient.

5. Charity-care provisions will be reevaluated for a patient's eligibility when the following occur:

- Subsequent rendering of services

- Income change

- Family size change

- When any part of the patient's account is written off as a bad debt or is in collections

- When six months have passed since the last application or when circumstances change, whichever comes first

6. Determine eligibility for charity service at the time of admission/pre-registration, or as soon as possible thereafter. In some cases, it can take investigation to determine eligibility, particularly when a patient has limited ability to provide needed information. Also, because of complications unforeseen at the time of admission, the patient may need to be reclassified as a full or partial charity.

7. Financial counselors, administration associates, and PFS staff can initiate the application process.

8. PFS account representatives will determine the write-off amount based on the aforementioned

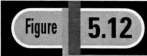

guidelines. If the patient does not meet the financial criteria but has extenuating circumstances such as catastrophic illness, the account will be referred to the supervisor who will make a recommendation to the director. Charity and discounted care approval authority is as follows:

- Write-offs from $.01 to $3,000 require approval by the appropriate PFS professional handling the account

- Write-offs from $3001 to $9,999 require approval by the PFS supervisor

- Write-offs from $10,000 to $24,999 require approval by the manager, PFS

- Write-offs $25,000 to $50,000 require approval by the director, PFS

- Write-offs greater than $50,000 require approval by the CFO

9. PFS staff will ensure that patients and physicians are notified, in writing, regarding approval, denial, or pending status of uncompensated care. The notification will include the appeal process for any denied application.

10. The appeal process for denied charity and discounted care applications includes the following activities:

- Prompt notification of the denial and the specific reasons will be provided to each charity and discounted care applicant. The notification will also provide examples of additional information, which may be used to appeal the denial.

- Additional information will be accepted by the provider, attached to the initial application, and routed to a designated manager for review.

- The denial reviewer will be a manager not involved in the initial determination process.

- If the initial denial is upheld, prompt notification will be provided to the patient. The patient will also be made aware of a final appeal opportunity.

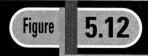

Detailed charity policy and procedures—Prototype document (cont.)

• The charity committee, acting as the CFO's designee for this process, will review all final appeals. A written determination will be issued within 15 days of the receipt of the final appeal.

Duties of the charity committee

11. Review all final denial applications for charity and discounted care, and re-determine eligibility based on established criteria. Suspend application when the patient should/has applied for Medicaid or Victims of Crime or has provided incomplete information. Ensure that all required documentation is provided.

12. Final denials may be appealed to the committee with the following documentation:

   • Appeal letter to committee from the patient or guarantor requesting reevaluation; appeal request from a PFS staff member

   • Supporting documents that may prove inability to pay that weren't part of the initial consideration

13. The committee will review appeals and the committee will make recommendations to the CFO or his designee for final approval.

Documentation retention and eligibility guidelines

14. The hospital will retain all charity and discounted care applications and supporting documentation for seven years.

15. The hospital will update the income eligibility criteria annually, using the federal poverty guidelines (FPG) published by the Centers for Medicare & Medicaid Services (CMS). If CMS issues more than one update, the updated criteria shall become effective as of the issue date.

16. As of "XX/XX/200X" the base level for the charity and discount care income eligibility will be set at "XXX%" of the current FPG.

Note: This policy and procedure is included on the accompanying CD-ROM.

Charity eligibility processing: Eligibility scales and forms

Income eligibility scales may be simple or complex; the same is true for the application form used by the provider. Complex eligibility scales typically reflect discounting to uninsured and underinsured patients in as few as four increments (discounts based on 25%, 50%, 75%, or 100% of charges) or as many as 10 (discounts ranging from 10% to 100% of charges, in 10% increments). Application forms need to be complex to the point of including both an income and asset test, but not so complex as to require hours of work to complete. Providers should review their applications periodically to make sure that they require only relevant information.

Figure	5.13	Amount of charity care determination based on 2004 federal poverty guidelines

Methodology: The Hospital uses the "Sliding Scale Method" to determine the dollar amount to be considered as charity care for eligible patients.

% FPL	Family size 1	2	3	4	5	6	7	8	Inpatient Pmt per day	ER services per visit	OP Surgery Per visit	Other O P Per visit
	Outpatient services payment											
100%	$9,310	$12,490	$15,670	$18,850	$22,030	$25,210	$28,390	$31,570	$	$	$	$
120%	$11,172	$14,988	$18,804	$22,620	$26,436	$30,252	$34,068	$37,884	$ 100	$ 35	$ 100	$ 35
140%	$13,034	$17,486	$21,938	$26,390	$30,842	$35,294	$39,746	$44,198	$ 200	$ 50	$ 200	$ 50
160%	$14,896	$19,984	$25,072	$30,160	$35,248	$40,336	$45,424	$50,512	$ 300	$ 65	$ 300	$ 65
180%	$16,758	$22,482	$28,206	$33,930	$39,654	$45,378	$51,102	$56,826	$ 400	$ 80	$ 400	$ 80
200%	$18,620	$24,980	$31,340	$37,700	$44,060	$50,420	$56,780	$63,140	$1,000	$ 120	$ 1,000	$ 120
220%	$20,482	$27,478	$34,474	$41,470	$48,466	$55,462	$62,458	$69,454	$1,050	$ 150	$ 1,050	$ 150
240%	$22,344	$29,976	$37,608	$45,240	$52,872	$60,504	$68,136	$75,768	$1,150	$ 175	$ 1,150	$ 175
260%	$24,206	$32,474	$40,742	$49,010	$57,278	$65,546	$73,814	$82,082	$1,250	$ 200	$ 1,250	$ 200
280%	$26,068	$34,972	$43,876	$52,780	$61,684	$70,588	$79,492	$88,396	$1,350	$ 250	$ 1,350	$ 250
300%	$27,930	$37,470	$47,010	$56,550	$66,090	$75,630	$85,170	$94,710	$1,450	$ 300	$ 1,450	$ 300
320%	$29,792	$39,968	$50,144	$60,320	$70,496	$80,672	$90,848	$101,024	$1,500	$ 325	$ 1,500	$ 325
340%	$31,654	$42,466	$53,278	$64,090	$74,902	$85,714	$96,526	$107,338	$1,550	$ 350	$ 1,550	$ 350
360%	$33,516	$44,964	$56,412	$67,860	$79,308	$90,756	$102,204	$113,652	$1,600	$ 375	$ 1,600	$ 375
380%	$35,378	$47,462	$59,546	$71,630	$83,714	$95,798	$107,882	$119,966	$1,650	$ 400	$ 1,650	$ 400
400%	$37,240	$49,960	$62,680	$75,400	$88,120	$100,840	$113,560	$126,280	$1,700	$ 450	$ 1,700	$ 450

Note: Another sample income eligibility chart was provided in Chapter 2. The complete instructions for updating that chart and the chart itself are included as an Excel file on the CD-ROM that accompanies this book.

The prototype application that follows is designed to collect all the information needed to process a charity and discounted care application. The provider adjudication section is specifically adapted to the eligibility chart displayed in this chapter. The complete application and sample letters are provided on the CD-ROM that accompanies this book. The adjudication section should be modified to provide a worksheet that mirrors the specific components of your charity and discounted services policy and procedures.

Figure 5.14 — Request for charity and discounted services form

As provided by hospital policy, I ask the Hospital to determine if I am eligible for help in paying for my hospital bill. I understand that I need to give certain information for this to be done. I also understand that these facts will be checked for accuracy by the Hospital or its agents. I understand that filling out this form does not guarantee that I will receive this help. If I am not eligible for charity or discounted services, I am responsible for my hospital bill.

Name _____ Account number _____
    First   Middle   Last

Address _____ Phone number ( ) _____
    Street   City   Zip

Employer name _____ Employer phone # _____

Employer address _____

Date of birth ___/___/___ Sex code ___ 1=Male 2= Female Social Security Number _____

Ethnicity: Enter ethnicity code as follows:

1	White	4	Asian
2	Black	5	Asian/Pacific Islander
3	Hispanic	6	Other

Last year of education completed _____
Number of family members living with you _
Name   Relationship   Age   Sex
_____
_____
_____
_____

Are you a U.S. citizen? _____ (1) Yes (2) No

Mother's maiden name _____
Place of birth   _____

FAMILY PRINCIPAL INCOME SOURCE:
Code _____

(01)	Professional/Technical
(02)	Labor/Production employment
(03)	Agricultural employment
(04)	Service/Sales employment
(05)	Unemployment compensation
(06)	Retirement income
(07)	Disability income
(08)	General relief
(09)	Other income source
(10)	None

Repeat patient?
Yes/No

Potential Third Party Payer Source
Code _____

(1)	Private insurance
(2)	Medicaid
(3)	Medicare
(4)	Self-pay
(5)	Other
(6)	None

Physician's name _____

Diagnosis _____

INCOME: PLEASE PROVIDE PHOTOCOPIES OF CHECKS AND
LIST INCOME FOR FAMILY FROM:

	Annual	Monthly
Wages (Self)		_____
(Spouse)		_____
(Other family member)		_____
Farm or self-employment		_____
Public assistance		_____
Social Security		_____
Unemployment compensation		_____
Strike benefits		_____

Figure 5.14 — **Request for charity and discounted services form (cont.)**

Alimony	_____
Child support	_____
Military family allotments	_____
Pensions	_____
Income from dividends, interest, rent	_____

ADDITIONALLY, PLEASE PROVIDE PHOTOCOPIES OF YOUR LAST TWO BANK STATEMENTS.

EXPENSES (Monthly)

Mortgage/Rent	_____ (1)	Medical insurance _____
Utilities	_____	Auto insurance _____
Telephone	_____	Medical bills _____
Food	_____	Hospital _____
Finance companies	_____	Physician_____
Credit union	_____	Medication _____
Auto loans	_____	

(1) If none, source of housing _____ TOTAL EXPENSES _____

Do you own a home?	Yes ( ) No ( )	If yes, estimated value: _____
Amount owed _____		
Do you own other property?	Yes ( ) No ( )	If yes, estimated value: _____
Do you own automobiles?	Yes ( ) No ( )	If yes, Model/Make Year Value

Bank references
Name/Branch _____   _____
Account #: _____   _____
Name/Branch _____   _____
Account #: _____   _____

- I declare under penalty of perjury that the answers I have given are true and correct to the best of my knowledge.
- I agree to tell the provider of services, within 10 days, if there are any changes in my (or the persons on whose behalf I am acting) income, property, expenses, or in the persons in the household, or of any changes of address.
- I understand that I may be asked to prove my statements and that my eligibility statements will be subject to verification by contact with my employer, bank, credit verification, and property searches.
- I understand that the county and hospital are required by law to keep any information I provide confidential.
- I further agree, that in consideration for receiving healthcare services as a result of an accident or injury, to reimburse the county or hospital from proceeds of any litigation or settlement resulting from such act.
- I understand that if I do not qualify for uncompensated services, I will be personally liable for the charges of the services rendered by the Hospital or I may appeal the decision in writing with additional documentation.

_____   _____
Signature   Date
_____   _____

FOR HOSPITAL USE ONLY:
LIABILITY COMPUTATIONS

Total Net Real and Personal Property Monthly Payment (A)	$_____
(+) Total Monthly Gross Income (B)	$_____
TOTAL MONTHLY INCOME	$_____
(-) Total Monthly Deductions (C)	$_____

Figure 5.14 Request for charity and discounted services form (cont.)

Type of service: Code: _____
(1) Hospital inpatient (2) Hospital outpatient (3) Hospital emergency room
Other qualified payer source, if any: _____
Units of service:

I/P Days billed amount	$_____	Approved _____	Date _____
Clinic visits	Payment collected $_____	Denied _____	Date ___
E/R visits	Other write-offs $_____	Pool log _____	Date ___
Admit date	_____	Patient liability _____	
Discharge date	_____		

Comments:
_____
_____
_____
_____

_____   _____
Signature   Date

Source: Sandra J. Wolfskill, FHFMA.

Sample system-generated notices

The use of system-generated notification letters to both patients and physicians accomplish the notification activity and ensure consistency in wording and message. These letters can be queued and completed as needed by the staff member processing the charity application. A copy of the letter is scanned into the patient's electronic financial folder for review, should the patient later file an appeal.

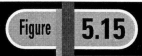

Sample system-generated notices

Patient notification letter

Date _____

Guarantor name _____

Patient name _____

Guarantor address _____

Patient's account number _____

Guarantor city, state, and ZIP code

_____

Date of service _____

Dear Mr./Mrs./Ms. _____,

We have carefully reviewed your application for charity and discounted care and have determined that your account

( )   meets the hospital's established guidelines for charity and discounted services.

( )   meets the hospital's established guidelines for charity and discounted services pending outcome/resolution of your Medicaid application/financial review.

100% charity care: Approved amount $_____.

Discounted care: Your account will be reduced by ____%, and the guarantor is responsible for $ _____.

You will be contacted within the next seven (7) days to establish payment terms for this amount.

( )   does not meet the hospital's established guidelines for charity and discounted services.

Figure	5.15	Sample system-generated notices (cont.)

Reason for denial:

_____ Monthly income exceeds qualifications

_____ Potential third-party payer source

_____ Application not complete

_____ Supporting documentation not adequate

If you wish to appeal this decision, please call _____ at _____
to initiate the appeal process.

Appeals must be filed within 10 days of the date of this letter.

Sincerely,

Patient Financial Services

Source: Sandra J. Wolfskill, FHFMA.

Figure	5.16	Sample notification to patient's physician

Physician name _____ Date _____

Date of service _____ Patient name _____

Patient's account number _____

Dear Doctor

We have carefully reviewed the application for charity and discounted care for your patient and have determined that your patient

( )   meets the hospital's established guidelines for charity and discounted services. We would like to ask you to consider extending charity and discounted services to this patient as well.

( )   meets the hospital's established guidelines for charity and discounted services pending outcome/resolution of the Medicaid application/financial review.

( )   does not meet the hospital's established guidelines for charity and discounted services.

Reason for denial:

_____   Monthly income exceeds qualifications

_____   Potential third party payer source

_____   Application not complete

_____   Supporting documentation not adequate

If you have questions, please call _____ at _____.

Sincerely,

Patient Financial Services

Summary

Best practices in revenue cycle management incorporate contemporary approaches to processing patient financial information. Making charity processing an integrated part of the pre-service and time of service activities recognizes the importance of providing patient financial education and resolving patient balances at the earliest appropriate opportunity. This approach ultimately reduces post-service work and leads to the correct classification of account write-offs identified as charity.

Implementing contemporary financial assistance policies and procedures

Implementing contemporary financial assistance policies and procedures

Getting started

Your organization's decision to change some or all of its processes related to charity care may be driven by several factors. The risk assessment (see Chapter 4) may have identified multiple opportunities for improvement. Your board of directors or finance committee may have read an article and raised probing questions concerning the current charity practices. A series of survey results may have raised significant patient satisfaction issues related to billing and collection, discounting, and charity. Regardless of why your organization needs to change its policies and procedures, as a revenue cycle professional, you are faced with changing your organization's charity and discounting practices.

The difficult decision is always where to start. How broken or dysfunctional are the current charity and discounting processes? Is the necessary change something as simple as revising the poverty guidelines, or are significant processes in need of revision? The degree of change will determine the scope of the project and the amount of resources realistically needed to achieve the desired results.

If the change is minor, then you do not need a formal work plan. You can prepare the change, obtain the needed approvals, and implement the process. For minor changes, only a minimal amount of staff training is required.

However, if process revisions are necessary, better planning will help you achieve positive results. Rushing headlong into making changes will not produce the desired results. Processes are interrelated, and patient financial services (PFS) does not operate in a vacuum. Often, process changes fail when the necessary parties are not involved and do not buy into the changes. Thus, getting started means building the case for change and presenting it to the right group within your organization.

The work plan

The work plan is a dynamic document used to track and control the project. The scope of the project determines the basic sections of the work plan. Use the plan to identify and assign individual projects and to post routine status updates. This single document not only lets the project team visually determine the status of the project, but it also tracks significant issues and roadblocks to completion. Every work plan will be different, though all work plans serve the same purpose: To document and track the project to ensure that all members of the project team are accountable for completing their part of it in a timely manner. In Figure 6.1, detailed tasks are only included for the initial section.

The project team

In project management, the "three Rs" do not refer to reading, writing, and arithmetic but to "right people," "right time," and "right size."

The "right people" refers to the inclusiveness of the project team. Financial operations do not occur separately from the clinical side of the organization. Clinicians are more likely to be supportive of a financial initiative when involved in it. Social workers are more likely to refer patients to financial counselors when both parties understand how their individual tasks support the organizational goal of appropriately resolving patient financial obligations in a timely manner. PFS staff are more likely to be excited about a project when line staff actively participate in project activities. Finally, the right administrative champion, who will take the project teams recommendations through the senior management approval process, is essential to the success of the project.

"Right time" refers to both the timing of the project in relation to other priorities already assigned to the management group and to the need to complete the project within a reasonable time. Clearly, the initiative to change charity processes must have a high priority and an adequate set of resources devoted to the project. Equally important, the project cannot become a never-ending series of meetings and conversations that produce no tangible results. The project team needs to be committed to devoting the time necessary to complete the assigned tasks within the project's life cycle.

Figure 6.1 — High-level project plan: Improvements in charity processing

ID #	Task description	Resp. party	Due date	% compl.	Status
A1.0	Administration • Select and recruit project team • Obtain administrative mandate • Determine project scope, objectives, and metrics • Establish tools (Intranet site for all documents, meeting agenda format, documentation rules, etc.) • Based on scope, identify initial target completion date • Schedule routine team meetings				
B1.0	Review of current state information				
C1.0	Development of best practice workflows				
D1.0	Development of policies and detailed procedures based on workflows				
E1.0	Identification and obtaining of system-based tools to support policies and procedures				
F1.0	Obtaining of approvals through administrative structure				
G1.0	Identification of resources and skill sets needed to implement new processes, including a staffing model, based on procedure requirements				
H1.0	Implementation of staffing development, including selection and training				
I1.0	Implementation and monitoring of changes				

Note: An Excel version of the complete prototype work plan document is included on the accompanying CD-ROM.

"Right size" refers to the concept of limits, both in terms of scope and in terms of team membership. A complete process redesign of the revenue cycle is a major undertaking requiring hundreds, if not thousands, of hours to complete. A project to restate the workflows and processes surrounding the resolution of charity and discounted care, however, is one subset of a major redesign effort. This smaller project is doable, which means that facilities can produce concrete results in a relatively short time (typically two to four months). Project planning focuses the team on the agenda at hand and helps to control the project, which can take on a life of its own, well beyond the original project charter. The size of the project team is also important. Facilities must balance the number of team members against the need to maintain current operations and the need to complete project activities in a timely manner. Having the right sized project team is essential to producing first-class results in the optimum amount of time.

Pre-service process

The typical project team for implementing changes to the charity and discounted care processes in the pre-service area should include staff and management from scheduling, ancillary services, patient access, patient financial counseling, patient accounts, and nursing.

Step one

The initial tasks should identify how the organization processes charity and discounted care applications and approvals before providing services. These tasks may include interviewing supervisors, managers, and staff, as well as observing work in the scheduling and financial counseling areas. Share the results of the risk and opportunity assessment with the project team.

Step two

Identify culture and customer service issues that adversely impact optimum performance in patient registration and patient accounts, and include these as issues to be resolved with the new workflows and procedures. For example, if a majority of the physicians' offices are not supportive of pre-service financial processing, develop education sessions presenting the case for this type of process. If customer service is not a priority among staff, Web-based customer service training can be developed and made available as the project develops.

Step three

Using best-practice workflows, the project team can develop the new, detailed workflows for the pre-service process. A production/exception model ensures that the team identifies and resolves all possible situations in an expedited manner. For example, the production activity may be to collect all financial information needed to resolve the charity and discounted care application during the initial financial education contact with the patient. Exceptions to this activity may include the following:

- The provider's inability to contact the patient prior to service

- The patient's inability to provide the required documents prior to service

- The patient's inability to understand what is being requested for the application

Step four

For each of these exceptions, the team should develop resolutions within the new workflows and procedures. Doing so ensures that standardized processing occurs, regardless of which member of the staff handles an account.

Step five

The team then identifies and prioritizes system needs and resources. The ability to distribute and control work using an automated system is critical to the success of pre-service processing. The use of a rules-based work distribution tool ensures that the organization achieves real-time movement of accounts based on required tasks and available resources.

Bolt-on technologies, such as a rules-based work distribution system, are ideal for this extension of the core scheduling, patient registration, and patient accounting systems. In this type of environment, the system queues scheduled patients for processing based on the type of insurance and managed care requirements. Once the system has determined and recorded the patient liability, the system workflow can then queue them so staff can contact and educate patients. Should charity screening be required, a separate workflow is established to control the charity process. If additional activity on the account by PFS staff is required, the rules-based work distribution system queues the account at the appropriate time. If the exception occurs (e.g., the charity process is not resolved prior to service), the system automatically triggers processing at the patient arrival checkpoint, which may be anywhere in the facility. This kind of system support eliminates manual work lists and ensures that the status of every scheduled patient's account is known in real-time.

Step six

Another important system tool for your team to develop is an online charity and discounted care application form. Deploying the application form on laptop computers enables financial counseling staff to complete the initial application at the bedside or point of service. Making the application form available on the provider's Web site with electronic submission also facilitates completion and return of the form.

Your team should also develop tools to help patients complete the financial aid application and screening. Develop a checklist geared to the specific requirements of the charity and discounted charges application to guide patients through the application process. See Figure 6.2 for a sample financial assistance checklist. A simple workflow creates a picture for the patient of what happens with the information and when the patient's application will be resolved. See Figure 6.3 for a sample application workflow. Making information—including application forms—available on your facility's Web site is another way to help support the process even before the patient arrives for service.

Scripting staff conversations with patients

Within the pre-service area, staff need to know how to discuss financial issues with patients. Scripting is a basic way that PFS directors can set the tone of each patient contact. It is also a way to eliminate the use of "hospital-speak" (i.e., jargon that is common to the healthcare industry). Scripting becomes a staff training tool that allows staff to practice in a classroom environment before actually implementing new procedures with patients.

To ensure a consistent approach, your team can develop a script for each common situation that staff may encounter. For example, one script may guide staff through the initial follow-up contact with the patient to provide financial education. In this contact, it is important to establish that this is not a collection call, but an information call. See Figure 6.4 for a sample script.

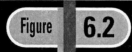

Figure 6.2

Sample patient checklist

ABC healthcare provider

Financial assistance checklist

The attached financial assistance application is our tool to determine your eligibility for charity and discounted care at our facility. You must complete this form and return it with copies of all the required documentation (see list). Items required for your specific application are marked with an "X." If we do not receive the completed application by the date specified, your application may be denied.

Financial assistance application must be returned by: _____

Application must be delivered to the Cashier's Office, Main Lobby, East Entrance, or mailed to: ABC Healthcare Provider, PO Box 111, Attn: PFS Dept., Anywhere, ST 11111.

Checklist of required information: (Copies only—no originals)

_____ Most recent bank statement for checking account

_____ Most recent bank statement for savings account

_____ Proof of income for the most recent three months

_____ Proof of income for the most recent 12 months

_____ Most recent income tax return

_____ Medicaid denial notice

_____ Unemployed—unemployment compensation determination or termination notice

_____ Prescription drug list

_____ Complete listing of all outstanding medical debt

Have you:

1. Completed the financial assistance application? _____

2. Have you signed the financial assistance application? _____

Please use this checklist to make sure your application is complete.

Please note that your signature verifies the accuracy of the information provided and authorizes ABC to verify any and all information provided.

Signature: _____

Note: This checklist is included on the CD-ROM accompanying this book.

Figure 6.3 — Sample application workflow illustration

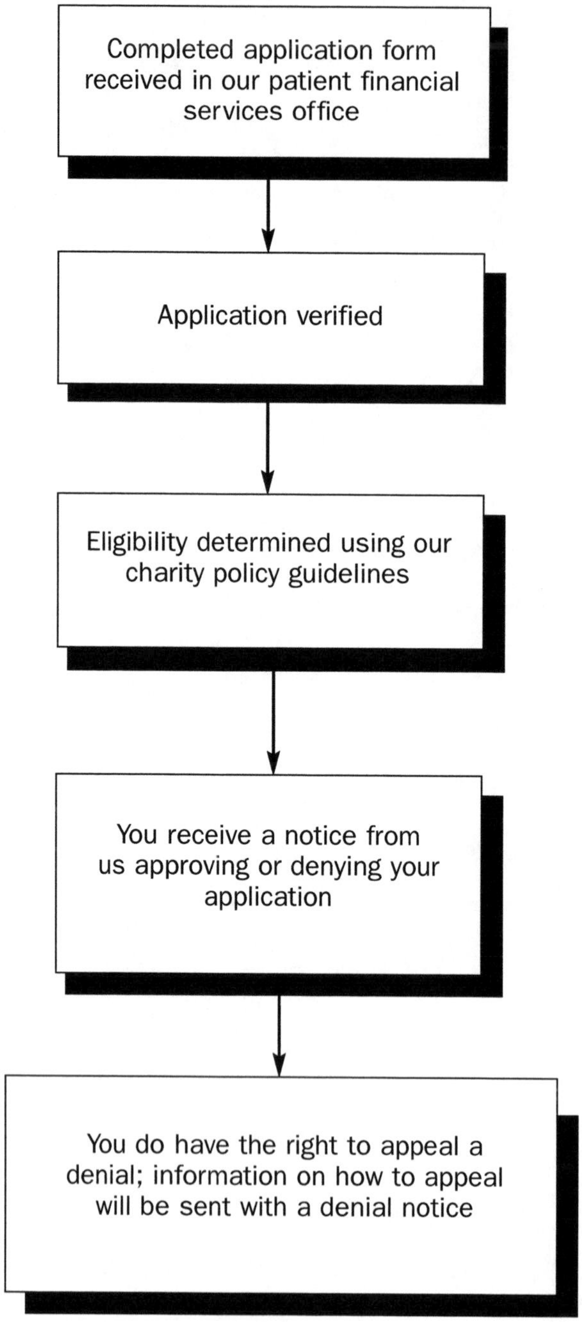

Completed application form received in our patient financial services office

↓

Application verified

↓

Eligibility determined using our charity policy guidelines

↓

You receive a notice from us approving or denying your application

↓

You do have the right to appeal a denial; information on how to appeal will be sent with a denial notice

| Figure | 6.4 | Sample script to provide patient education and initiate charity processing |

PFS staff: Good morning/afternoon/evening. My name is Carol, and I am calling from ABC Provider to speak with Mrs. Smith.

Mrs. Smith: Yes, this is Mrs. Smith.

PFS staff: Mrs. Smith, may I have your date of birth for identification purposes?

Mrs. Smith: *Provides date of birth*

PFS staff: Thank you. Mrs. Smith, the reason I am calling you today is to share with you the information we have collected concerning your insurance benefits for your upcoming service. Is this a good time for us to talk?

If response is yes:

PFS staff: Thank you. We have checked with XZY Benefits, your insurance company, and learned that your coverage has been terminated. Have you obtained other insurance?

Mrs. Smith: No, my husband has been unemployed now for almost six months and we do not have insurance.

PFS staff: Mrs. Smith, I am sorry to hear that. If you qualify, our hospital has a program to help patients with their hospital bills. May I tell you about this program?

Mrs. Smith: Yes, please do.

The staff member goes on to explain the financial assistance program in easy-to-understand terms. This scripting provides a guide to the explanation and leads the staff member into completing a preliminary application over the telephone. Based on the income and other information provided, PFS staff give a preliminary eligibility indication to the patient and explain the documentation requirements for final approval. The script goes on to tell the patient that the facility will mail a copy of the application information and requirements today or, if the service is scheduled within three days, that the application will be available when he or she arrives for the service.

If the patient says this is not a good time to talk, the script guides the staff member through identifying a time to schedule the return call, closes the conversation by thanking the patient for his or her time, and reminds the patient about the scheduled return call.

Staffing requirements

Process redesign and revision fails when the organization does not objectively identify the staffing requirements needed to support the redesigned processes. Only after completing the workflows and policies and procedures and identifying the activity volumes can facilities accurately determine staffing levels. For example, if the facility adds patient financial education as a new activity for pre-service processing, there is a staffing requirement associated with that activity. To determine the full-time equivalent (FTE) requirements for the redesigned pre-service process, use the following steps:

1. Identify the annual volumes for each activity in the process.

2. Determine the average amount of time needed to complete each activity.

3. Multiply the volumes by the times to determine the total time required annually.

4. Add up the hours required for each position in the department.

5. Complete the calculation by converting the time into hours, then divide that number by your FTE equivalent factor to determine the FTEs required.

See Figure 6.5 for a sample FTE calculation.

Staffing the new process

In addition to determining the number of staff required, the new position descriptions need to identify clearly the skills needed for each position. Once the facility has confirmed the number of staff required, approved the position descriptions, and resolved the staff redeployment process, the hospital may post and fill the positions according to policy.

Necessary training

Once staff have been selected/added, depending on the amount of change necessitated by the redesign, training becomes a major activity. To be effective, training should be provided "just in time" (i.e., just before the actual implementation of the new processes, not three or four weeks in advance) in formal classroom sessions, complete with handout materials, copies of the new procedures, workflows, and scripts. Each class should also include ample time for staff to practice the scripts until they achieve a comfort level.

Figure 6.5	Sample FTE calculation for a pre-service financial counseling area						
Activity	**Volume statistic FY 2004**	**Current process time required**	**Process redesign time required (in minutes)**	**New process time x volume calc**	**Process redesign calculated process FTEs—productive**	**Process redesign calculated process FTEs—non-productive**	**Comments**
Insurance	158,500	2	2	317,000			100% verification; electronic
Managed care	71,325	6	6	427,950			45% penetration
Anticipate charges and calculate patient liability	110,950	5	5	554,750			
Apply benefits	110,950	2	2	221,900			Historic data: 70% of patients owe portion
Contact patient—financial education	110,950	7	7	776,650			
Charity application initiate	11,095	n/a	10	110,950			Est. 10% of patients may qualify; 12% non-productive time per payroll
Totals				2,409,200	19.3	2.6	
Total for area						**21.9**	

Note: This worksheet is included on the accompanying CD-ROM.

All employees need to have a basic understanding about the revised charity processes. Although the training does not need to be as detailed for all employees as it is for the PFS staff, awareness leads to support, which translates into a positive image of the new processes for the staff and the community.

Performance metrics

Finally, the project team needs to establish performance metrics and measurement systems to monitor the redesigned processes. Without measurement and statistics, facilities cannot identify and celebrate successes or recognize shortfalls. For example, your facility may set the initial metric for completion of charity applications prior to service at 25% of the patients identified as potentially eligible for charity service. However, three months after implementing the process change, the metric changes to 50%, and six months after implementation, the expected performance may be 85% of the patients in this category.

Thus, the metrics established in one area, especially if incremental standards are used, must be coordinated across process areas. The best approach is to develop the entire performance measurement package at one time, before staff training and implementation. A significant use of performance measurement is to monitor staff productivity and performance. For example, a productivity measure may be defined as 100% of scheduled patients who are identified as potential charity cases are resolved (approved or denied) no later than time of service. Another metric may be that 100% of charity applications are correctly approved or denied. Regardless of which metrics you use, to be effective, staff need to understand the measurement expectations and calculations.

Time-of-service process

Time-of-service processing includes two groups of patients: those scheduled and those not scheduled for service. For the scheduled patient, this phase of the revenue cycle involves patient arrival processing and provision of service. For the unscheduled patient, this phase includes all activities required to process a patient, including registration, insurance verification, managed care resolution, medical necessity screening, charge anticipation, financial education, resolution, and provision of clinical services.

If the organization has revised the pre-service process for scheduled patients to include charity processing, the impact on the time-of-service process will vary based on the scheduled or unscheduled status of the patient. For scheduled patients, the charity process may be limited to collecting copies of documents and obtaining the patient's signature on the printed application form. For unscheduled patients, however, there may be significant process changes.

Step one

Within the unscheduled patient population, the provider may elect to establish thresholds for completing financial education and counseling. The project team collects data and determines where the effort costs more than the benefit received by the organization. Examples of data reviewed include average dollar value of unscheduled tests (such as laboratory tests), average numbers of unscheduled patients by service area, service area denial information, and bad debts by service area. The project team also recognizes for example, that, based on best-practice models, the patient flow in the emergency department (ED) requires major revisions and close coordination between the clinical and PFS staff.

Step two

Some members of the pre-service team typically join the time-of-service discussions. Their involvement ensures that there are no gaps between what is planned before the service and what occurs when the patient arrives at the facility. Whereas scheduling and registration staff may serve on the pre-service team, the time-of-service team typically adds ED staff to the project team.

Step three

The initial tasks on the project plan should focus on identifying the process used by the pre-service team. Based on this model, the team will need to identify what they need to accomplish at the time of service. Be sure to share the results of the risk assessment with the project team.

Step four

Identify culture and customer-service issues that adversely impact optimum performance and include these as issues to resolve using the new workflows and procedures. For example, if a majority of ED nurses and physicians oppose financial discharge processing, the team can develop education sessions presenting the case for this type of process. If customer service is not a priority among staff, Web-based customer service training can be made available as the project develops.

Step five

Using best practice workflows, the project team develops the new, detailed workflows for the time of service. A production/exception model ensures that all possible situations are identified and resolved in an expedited manner. For example, the production activity in time-of-service processing is to complete a registration for the unscheduled patient at the time of service. An exception to this activity would be that services were provided before the registration activity was completed; in such a case, the registration activity must be completed at a later point in the process. Another example of an exception would be an incomplete charity application initiated during the pre-service process. The resolution of this activity is that the patient needs to provide supporting documentation and sign the charity application at the time of service. The final part of the resolution process consists of scanning the documents into the patient's electronic financial record, obtaining the patient's signature on the printed application form, and providing the financial counseling required based on the eligibility determination.

Step six

The system tools discussed in the pre-service section of this chapter are equally important to the time-of-service processing for charity care. In addition to controlling the required workflows for unscheduled patients, the rules-based application can help patient-access staff complete the remaining requirements for the scheduled patients at the desktop, without relying on lists or paper reports.

Facilities can use the same checklist (Figure 6.2) to help the patient complete the charity application with all applications distributed at the time of service. In addition, the facility can provide stamped, self-addressed return envelopes to expedite the return of the completed application and supporting documentation.

Scripting staff conversations with patients

Scripting is equally important for time-of-service issues. Many of the scripts developed for use in the pre-service area are easily adapted to the time-of-service setting. A complete set of scripts for the emergency-department discharge process and financial education/charity processing is included on the CD-ROM with this book.

Staffing requirements

Once the complete time-of-service activities for charity processing have been determined, facilities can apply the same staffing methodology used for the pre-service activities to the time-of-service processes. Typically, staffing increases occur in the financial counseling areas and in the ED discharge processing area.

Staffing the new process

In addition to determining the number of staff required, the new position descriptions need to identify clearly the skills needed for each position. Once the facility has confirmed the number of staff required, approved the position descriptions, and resolved the staff redeployment process, the hospital may post and fill the positions according to policy.

Necessary training

Training for the time-of-service process changes follows the same track as the pre-service training. Specific materials are developed and used for PFS staff by the project team. In addition, organization-wide updates should be provided to all employees to gain a positive reaction to the redesigned process-es. These updates may be provided through newsletter articles, through bulletins on the hospital's intranet, or at department meetings.

Performance metrics

Performance metrics for the time-of-service areas will include a set of metrics and performance expectations for the unscheduled patients that are similar to those established in the pre-service process. Additional metrics will be needed to complete charity processing initiated but not fully resolved prior to the service.

Post-service process

The typical project team for implementing post-service changes to the charity process should include several individuals familiar with the redesigned pre-service and time-of-service processes, as well as staff from the customer service and collections areas. If the facility uses an outsource vendor for self-pay processing, invite that vendor to join the team. Finally, although the facility's collection agencies do not need to participate on the project team, they need to understand the provider's changes and expectations for accurate classification of accounts, even when delinquent collection activity is involved.

Culturally, charity process change involves convincing patient accounts staff that financial counselors and others in the access areas can process and approve charity applications accurately and appropriately. One tip for reducing the adverse reaction to such change is to reallocate those experienced patient accounts staff into the access areas.

Step one

The post-service team will need to understand all redesigned workflows and the policies and procedures created by the pre-service and time-of-service teams. The critical task for the post-service team is to ensure that staff properly screen every patient and that the facility only sends true bad debt accounts to collection agencies for additional processing.

Step two

Production/exception processing is also appropriate for the post-service charity processes. A production activity in post-service processing is to complete a charity application for a newly identified, potential charity case. The exception is when the patient returns the application that is not signed and dated. In this case, the resolution involves contacting the patient and obtaining the required signature. Post-service processes will typically focus on newly identified charity cases and exceptions from earlier phases of the charity process. This team must review carefully the detailed charity processes already designed and use their experience to capture all possible charity-related activities.

Step three

The same rules-based system tools discussed in earlier sections of this chapter are essential to track the next activity for incomplete charity applications and to initiate charity processing for newly identified charity cases. Work queues may be used to track incomplete applications, appeals, and individual parts of the charity approval process. Facilities can configure the same work-distribution application used in the pre-service and time-of-service areas to support the post-service processing requirements.

Scripting staff conversations with patients

Facilities can use the same scripts developed to support charity process changes in other phases of the revenue cycle in the post-service arena. Some modification may be needed to establish processing deadlines, etc.

Staffing requirements

Staffing calculations for the post-service charity process changes use the same model as previously discussed. Typically, staffing reductions may occur in the post-service area, which makes personnel available for pre-service or time-of-service processing. In other cases, additional tasks, such as contacting patients by telephone to complete the charity application, may be added in this area.

Staffing the new process

However, a staffing requirements review is still needed to determine the number of staff required, and the new position descriptions need to identify clearly the skills needed for each position. Once the facility has confirmed the number of staff required, approved the position descriptions, and resolved the staff redeployment process, the hospital may post and fill the positions according to policy.

Necessary training

Training requirements are minimal in the post-service implementation because staff are typically trained in their new work areas (i.e., pre-service or time-of-service).

Performance metrics

Performance metrics in the post-service implementation focus on accurate and complete resolution of all charity applications and adjustments.

Communicating with patients and physicians

No charity process is complete without communicating with the applicant (i.e., the patient) and the patient's physician, especially if the physician has been involved in requesting a charity consideration or if the physician is part of an integrated delivery system owned by the hospital. This communication needs to be timely and distributed in a way that protects the patient's privacy.

Communication with patients: The patient-friendly billing project approach

One of the major challenges in charity-care processing is communicating with patients in clear, understandable terms. The Healthcare Financial Management Association (HFMA) Patient Friendly Billing project has published a series of FAQs that apply to charity processing as well as to other billing and collection activities in the healthcare revenue cycle. For the complete description of this project, access HFMA's Web site at *www.hfma.org*.

As part of the implementation process, consider answering these questions for any patient inquiring about charity care:

1. How much will I really owe?
2. Who can I call for help?
3. Where are your offices located?
4. If I have other questions about my bill, who do I call?
5. How long will it take you to review my charity application?
6. What happens if you deny my application and I cannot pay my bill?
7. Can I get a copy of the charity application on the Internet?
8. For how long is my charity approval valid?

Develop a brochure designed to promote charity care and answer these common questions. By making the process easier to understand, you may increase your charity write-offs and reduce the bad debt losses.

Communication with physicians

Patients often communicate their frustrations and concerns about a hospital's billing and collection practices with their physician instead of with the hospital. Therefore, it is important that your facility share information with physicians and their office staff as you develop major changes in the facility's charity processes. A brief presentation at a medical staff meeting and a luncheon of physician office staff, complete with handouts and brochures, are effective communication tools.

Outsourcing charity processing

Although providers do not typically outsource charity processing by itself, there are opportunities in the contemporary environment to include charity application processing in a self-pay outsourcing program. As an alternative to implementing a complete in-house charity processing program, a provider may opt to outsource self-pay processing as soon as the account is identified as self-pay. This may occur during pre-registration or registration, or after the patient's insurance has paid. If the provider elects to outsource all self-pay processing, then including charity as part of the outsourced work is an excellent technique. By allowing the outsource vendor to handle not only the collection of self-pay dollars but, more importantly, the complete and appropriate resolution of self-pay accounts, you ensure consistency in the application of the provider's required processes. With this type of program, the outsource vendor assumes responsibility for providing charity applications, collecting the supporting documentation, and recommending the disposition of the application based on the eligibility criteria provided by the provider. The provider retains responsibility for final review and adjustment processing. The more progressive self-pay outsource vendors provide this service to their clients at no charge, as a value-added service.

Summary

Changing charity processes requires a disciplined approach and a team effort. The more significant the change, the greater the effort. However, the rewards include improved patient satisfaction and more appropriate classification of charity and bad debt dollars.

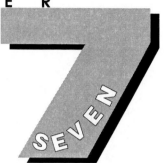

Case studies

Case studies

Providers have taken a variety of approaches to improving and expanding charity processing within their organizations. The case studies selected for this chapter represent three different providers:

- Camden-Clark Memorial Hospital (CCMH)—a 313-bed community hospital located in Parkersburg, WV

- "Hospital"—a 586-bed healthcare system, located in a two-hospital midwestern city

- West Virginia University Hospitals (WVUH) and University Health Associates (UHA)—a 522-bed hospital and a university faculty practice with 417,000 annual patient visits, located in Morgantown, WV

For each provider, we conducted an Internet search of their Web sites to provide basic information about each facility and to illustrate the different amounts of billing and charity-care information provided to the general public.

There are differences among the three cases, but the common thread is a willingness to expand eligibility criteria and to make the charity and discounting options work for their patient populations.

Case study 1: Camden-Clark Memorial Hospital

Provider Internet profile

"As the community's hospital for more than a century, Camden-Clark has always been committed to providing the best in healthcare. Since our founding in 1898, Camden-Clark Memorial Hospital has provided the finest possible healthcare to the people of our community. Our 1,450 employees, 200 medical staff, and over 550 Auxilians and hospital volunteers are dedicated to bringing every patient the care and attention necessary for a successful recovery."[1]

Uncompensated care information

None provided on Web site.

Figure 7.1	Camden-Clark's statistical profile
Annual net revenue	$136,838,941
Provider type	Community hospital
Bed size	313
Governance	Nonprofit
Bad Debt as % of net revenue (FY04)	7%
Charity as % of net revenue (FY04)	3%

Charity-care issues

The patient financial services (PFS) department recently completed an extensive review and redesign of the hospital's revenue cycle. With this review came the opportunity to make changes to existing policies and procedures. One policy that needed a major overhaul was the charity-care policy.

The existing policy was not meeting the patients' needs and did not allow for realistic account resolution. Frequently, patients did not meet CCMH's charity-care guidelines but were unable to pay the account in a reasonable amount of time. The timing of the financial counseling activity was also an issue. Patients would leave the hospital and receive one or more bills before the hospital discovered the patient's need for financial assistance.

Charity-processing changes

CCMH recognized that it had to apply uniformly its financial assistance program in order to provide financial help to those who qualify for it. The key to administering a charity program effectively starts before the patient ever presents for service.

The hospital included pre-registration and financial resolution prior to service in the redesigned process. However, because there will always be cases that require intervention and resolution after the provision of service, CCMH realized that it needed to use strategies to motivate patient participation in the account resolution process.

First, CCMH revised the charity-care guidelines using the federal poverty guidelines (FPG) as the baseline and incorporating a sliding scale approach. Patients with incomes at or below 200% of the FPG are eligible for a 100% bill adjustment, if they have no insurance coverage, or after insurance payment, if the patient has coverage. The hospital also considers the patient's household net monthly income and available assets. Those patients not qualifying for the 100% adjustment may be eligible for a 25%, 50%, or 75% bill adjustment, according to the sliding scale. The hospital then establishes payment arrangements for the remaining balance.

Second, the hospital created an Excel-based application form that records the information provided by the patient. Upon completion of the application form, the hospital can print the form and deliver it to the patient so the patient can sign it and attach proof of income. This automated tool has eliminated inconsistencies and allowed CCMH to include charity processing in the outsourcing contract with their outsourcing partner. A copy of the application form is included on the accompanying CD-ROM.

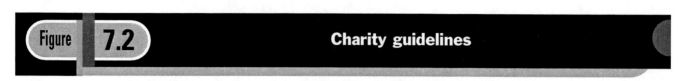

CCMH charity income eligibility scale updated to 2005 FPG

Size of family unit	Federal poverty guidelines	200%	201% - 250%			251% - 300%			301% - 350%		
1	9,570	19,140	19,141	-	23,925	23,926	-	28,710	28,711	-	33,495
2	12,830	25,660	25,661	-	32,075	32,076	-	38,490	38,491	-	44,905
3	16,090	32,180	32,181	-	40,225	40,226	-	48,270	48,271	-	56,315
4	19,350	38,700	38,701	-	48,375	48,376	-	58,050	58,051	-	67,725
5	22,610	45,220	45,221	-	56,525	56,526	-	67,830	67,831	-	79,135
6	25,870	51,740	51,741	-	64,675	64,676	-	77,610	77,611	-	90,545
7	29,130	58,260	58,261	-	72,825	72,826	-	87,390	87,391	-	101,955
8	32,390	64,780	64,781	-	80,975	80,976	-	97,170	97,171	-	113,365
Each additional person add	3,260	6,520	8,150			9,780			11,410		
Net monthly expenses/single		400	500			600			700		
Eeach additional person add		200	250			300			350		
Allowable assets		8,000	10,000			12,000			14,000		
Amount eligible for charity write-off		100% of balance	75% of balance			50% of balance			25% of balance		

Third, CCMH revised the financial counseling procedures and hired staff to perform financial counseling prior to the patient's date of service or on the day of service before the patient leaves the facility. The results have been positive. Patients say they appreciate the opportunity to discuss their financial obligations before having services.

Finally, during the redesign project, studies indicated that the hospital's volume of self-pay receivables was too great for the staff to manage effectively. The hospital decided to outsource the self-pay processing. Unlike the more traditional "Day 30" or "Day 45" outsourcing programs, CCMH selected a program that outsourced self-pay accounts on Day 1. The charity-care program and financial counseling continues with their outsourcing partner's staff. If the patient's circumstances did not allow for financial counseling prior to the patient's departure from the facility, the hospital uses the same procedures during the outsourced follow-up process.

Impact of changes

Within the first month of implementing the new processes (e.g., proactive financial counseling, revised charity eligibility scale, and outsourcing self-pay accounts), the hospital has increased the amount of charity provided.

The outsource partner also brought a new and patient-focused philosophy to the charity component of CCMH's revenue cycle process. When working with patients and helping them resolve their accounts, the goal should always be to identify where the patient falls in the "ability to pay" v. "willingness to pay" matrix. By asking open-ended questions, staff first identify whether the patient has the ability to pay the account, based on the options provided by CCMH. These payment options include a credit card or check payment, a hospital-sponsored low-interest medical loan, or in-house payment plan. For those

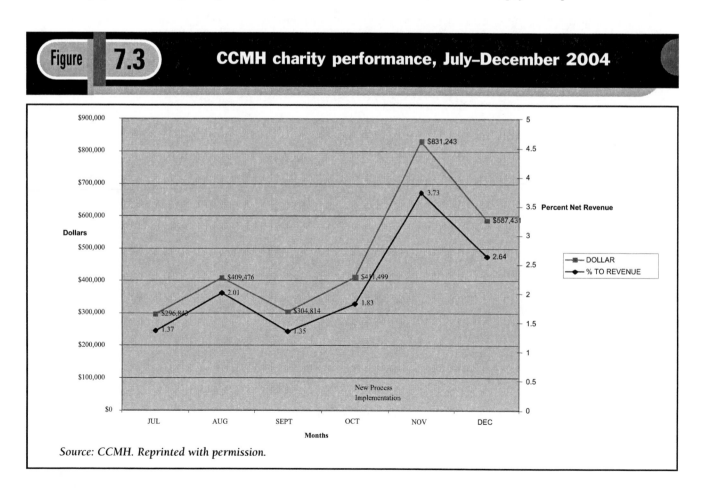

Figure 7.3 **CCMH charity performance, July–December 2004**

Source: CCMH. Reprinted with permission.

patients with the ability and willingness to pay, resolution of the account becomes a straightforward activity. However, a certain percentage of the patient population includes patients who have the means to pay the account but, for a variety of reasons, refuse to be compliant. For those situations, the services of a licensed collection agency are appropriate.

For the most part, patients are grateful for the care they receive and want to pay their bills. With the changing demographics of the average self-pay account, not all patients find themselves in a position to fully compensate the hospital for its services; this holds true regardless of whether they are willing to pay. This is where the revised charity policy came into play for CCMH.

The outsourcing vendor also taught CCMH the following:

> One of the keys in getting patients to cooperate with your data requests required to qualify for charity is always keeping their dignity intact and providing an environment that fosters a desire on their part to help the hospital in getting their account resolved. If you take an aggressive collection stance at the beginning of the patient contact, only to find out the patient does not have the ability to pay, their desire to help may be reduced. On the other hand, if you show care and empathy and demonstrate you are there to help them, not just collect money, their desire and willingness to provide the documentation necessary to comply with your charity policy is greatly increased.[2]

As a result, when a patient calls concerning his or her bill and staff identify the appropriateness of charity, the outsourcing vendor initiates the charity application on the telephone with the patient. The vendor arranges a callback time that allows the patient the opportunity to collect the needed documentation of income and assets. The vendor completes the application, prints and mails it to the patient with instructions to sign the form, attaches the proof-of-income documents, and mails the form to the hospital for final approval. The application form automatically calculates the patient's eligibility based on the current eligibility chart used by CCMH. Thus, the hospital does not face the patient with a complex application to complete, and he or she knows the results of the eligibility screening immediately. The outsource vendor will complete the approval process, including all notifications of approvals and denials to the patient, and submit the completed packet to CCMH for approvals based on the dollar amount of the charity adjustment.

Although CCMH is in the early stages of these process changes, it has already experienced positive results. The staff is pleased with the opportunity for early account resolution. Patients have provided positive feedback regarding the up-front financial counseling, particularly those patients scheduled for outpatient surgery or an extensive procedure that may result in a substantial bill. Outsourcing the self-pay receivable allows a dedicated resource to work effectively with the patients to resolve account balances and allows CCMH staff the time they need to focus on insurance receivables.

Case study 2: 'Hospital'—regional medical center

Provider Internet profile

"[Hospital] is an integrated healthcare system serving a 14-county area in the Midwest. [Hospital] is a 586-bed acute care center that provides inpatient, outpatient, and a variety of community outreach services. Hospital is the first and only hospital in its region to use a new cardiovascular digital imaging system in its cardiac catheterization lab and the only hospital in its county with a Level III neonatal intensive care unit."

Uncompensated care information from the Web site

"For generations, [Hospital] has provided its patients the highest quality of healthcare services. At [Hospital] every person receiving care is accorded the same rights and is treated with the same high level of dignity and respect regardless of ability to pay.

We understand hospital services can create financial concerns for you. We are prepared to help you by discussing your payment options for hospital services not covered by insurance (such as deductibles, copayments, or non-covered services). These amounts may be paid when you are dismissed from [Hospital].

For patients expressing an inability to pay, it is very important that you call one of our customer service representatives as soon as possible so we can start the review of your financial situation. Depending on your financial situation, you may qualify for Medicaid or our financial assistance program."[3]

Figure 7.4	Hospital statistical profile
Annual net revenue	$409,834,000
Provider type	Community hospital
Bed size	506
Governance	Nonprofit
Bad debt as % of net revenue (FYXX)	3%
Charity as % of net revenue (FYXX)	1.6%

Charity-care issues

The national attention to charity and discounted care and the American Hospital Association guidance to hospitals on the subject convinced PFS management to initiate significant changes to the charity practices.

Charity processing changes

Under the previous charity policy, charity was extended to patients whose income was up to 150% of the FPG. No discounts were provided except those negotiated by third-party payers. The workflow in Figure 7.5 illustrates the old and the new charity processes:

In addition to revising the basic charity workflow, Hospital revised three major policies and procedures: the core financial policy, the financial assistance policy, and the discounted care policy.

Provider forms

Hospital also developed two forms to use in the new charity process. First, the hospital uses a control sheet (i.e., placement worksheet) to document the movement of the accounts through the approval process. A sample worksheet is included on the accompanying CD-ROM. The second form

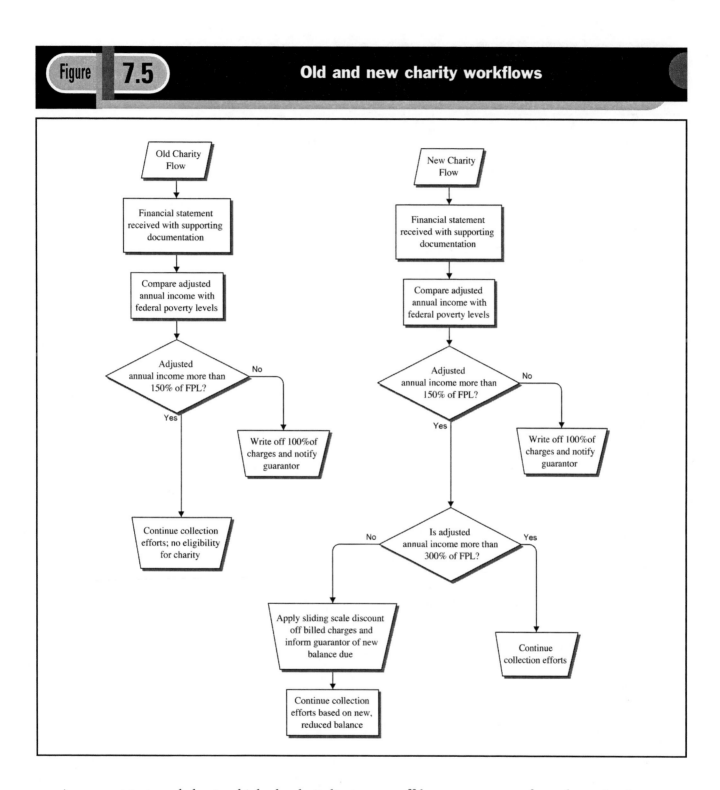

Figure 7.5 — **Old and new charity workflows**

is an asset test worksheet, which clearly indicates to staff how to use assets from the patient's federal income tax return in the income eligibility determination. A sample of this worksheet is also included on the CD-ROM.

Figure 7.6   Accounts receivable financial policy

Purpose: To ensure a consistent method of determining a patient's ability to pay and provide a process for financial resolution of accounts receivable.

Comprehensive access processing: Comprehensive access processing includes the collection and verification of the comprehensive data set, insurance eligibility and benefit verification, managed care requirement resolutions, charge anticipation, and calculation of patient and third-party liability including unresolved preexisting balances, financial education, and financial resolution.

Threshold determination: Thresholds are utilized where processing volumes prevent the ability to complete comprehensive access processing for 100% of patients. Threshold processing according to established procedure will be utilized based on charge criteria, patient liability criteria, and services identified where reimbursement would be affected without comprehensive processing.

Emergency medical conditions: Hospital will treat all patients with emergency medical conditions, as defined by COBRA/EMTALA regulations, regardless of their ability to pay. Emergency patients will be registered by obtaining the emergency data set as a minimum with the goal of obtaining and verifying the comprehensive data set and completing comprehensive access processing within the next business day.

Non-emergency medical conditions: Hospital will obtain and verify the comprehensive data set and complete comprehensive access processing for all non-emergency patients that meet threshold requirements prior to service for scheduled patients and at the time of service for non-scheduled patients. A minimum data set as established by Hospital will be required prior to scheduled finalization for all scheduled patients.

Financial resolution options: Financial resolution options based on requested service:

1. Elective non-covered surgery (i.e., cosmetic surgery, tubal reversal, etc.)

    • Full payment of patient liability prior to service, unless surgery is covered under a policy that allows a specific down payment prior to service

    • Services will be postponed or canceled until payment can be made

Figure 7.6 — Accounts receivable financial policy (cont.)

2. Medically necessary services that meet threshold criteria

- For identified non-authorized (non-preauthorized, non-precertified, or out-of-network) services for scheduled patients and non-scheduled invasive procedures, the physician will be contacted to obtain authorization or review service alternatives. If pre-authorization/pre-certification cannot be obtained, the patient will be given the option of rescheduling the procedure.

- The identified patient liabilities exceeding established thresholds will be requested during pre-service or at time of service, using payment options including cash, check, debit card, or credit card. Credit and debit cards will be accepted upon verification.

3. Patients stating an inability to pay will be referred for alternative program eligibility screening including Medicaid, payment plans, and financial assistance based on established financial screening criteria.

Third-party financial liabilities: Hospital will accept assigned benefits once the insurance has been verified. This does not relieve the patient of his or her financial liabilities, and the patient will be sent a status update regarding the status of each account, except where prohibited by federal regulations or contract (e.g., Medicaid). Insurance follow-up will be initiated according to a payer's established clean-claim payment cycle. Insurance accounts remaining unresolved 30 days beyond the clean-claim payment cycle will revert to the patient to satisfy the financial liabilities, except where prohibited by contract.

Patient financial liabilities: Patients without insurance or proof of insurance will be registered as self-pay and referred for financial counseling and Medicaid eligibility screening. Statements will be sent no less than monthly for patient financial liabilities and unresolved open balances will be referred for further action when the account has aged no more than 90 days from the initial bill date. Hospital or designee will authorize the filing of liens to recover patient financial liabilities.

Discounting services: Discounts on services rendered by Hospital are extended as a result of negotiated contracts with employers or third-party networks. The patient identification card must be current and clearly identify the network accessing Hospital services and discounts. It is the responsibility of

Figure 7.6   **Accounts receivable financial policy (cont.)**

payers and/or patients to make Hospital aware of the desire to use a specific contract and show cause that we should honor it at the time of benefit confirmation. Discounts claimed by the patient's insurance provider at time of payment that were not claimed at the time of service will be denied.

Financial assistance program: Hospital will provide financial assistance to qualifying patients who are U.S. citizens and have resided in this state for at least six months. Account balances will be forgiven for qualifying patients with an income level at or below 150% of the current Department of Health and Human Services federal poverty guidelines. For qualifying patients without health insurance who have an income level from 151% to 300% of the poverty guidelines, a sliding scale discount off charges will be provided. Patients requesting financial assistance are required to complete the established financial statement form and will be screened to verify eligibility according to an established procedure.

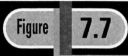

Figure 7.7 — Financial assistance determination procedure #10-20f

Department: Pre-access services and patient financial services (PFS)

Policy: Patients expressing an inability to pay for medically necessary services at Hospital will be asked to complete a financial statement application form so they can be evaluated for financial assistance under the accounts receivable financial policy. Eligible patients completing the application and providing all the requested information verifying their income and assets will be evaluated for eligibility for financial assistance. However, patients who have been referred to the Hospital assistance program and refused to cooperate or seek alternate resources will not be eligible for financial assistance and will not be sent a financial statement to complete.

Purpose: To provide a consistent process for evaluating patients for the Hospital financial assistance program.

Procedure:

1. Obtain completed financial statement and all pertinent attachments according to application instructions.

2. Verify Medicaid eligibility with EDS Web site (Medicaid eligibility files).

3. If the patient does not have Medicaid eligibility, attach a screen print of this to the financial statement and proceed to step four.

   - If the patient has Medicaid eligibility, add this information to the patient's account and order a single bill request. The patient no longer needs to be considered for financial assistance.

4. Examine and determine authenticity of attachments (e.g., pay stubs, U.S. tax return, notarized documents, etc.).

5. Verify financial information and medical information entries with documentation.

6. Determine patient's adjusted annual income from information provided on financial statement.

   - Multiply total monthly income by 12 to compute total yearly income.

**Financial assistance determination procedure
#10-20f (cont.)**

- Multiply monthly insurance premium and prescription drugs monthly by 12 to compute yearly amounts; then add Hospital bills, affiliated clinic bills, yearly amounts for insurance premiums, and yearly prescription drugs to determine total yearly medical information.

- Subtract total medical information from total yearly income. This is the adjusted annual income.

7. Using adjusted annual income, compare the number of persons supported by total monthly income (verified by the income tax return) with income level guidelines.

- If the adjusted annual income amount determined by step five is *below* the income level listed by the appropriate family size and the amounts on the patients income tax return do not exceed the income thresholds, the patient is eligible for financial assistance. Go to step eight.

- If the adjusted annual income amount determined by step five is *above* the income level listed by the appropriate family size, the patient does not qualify for financial assistance. Refer to policy #10-20d Payment Plan Resolution.

- If the adjusted annual income amount determined by step five is *below* the income level listed by the appropriate family size, *but* the amounts on the patient's income tax return exceed the threshold, send the patient a request for additional financial information letter requesting most recent statements for checking, saving accounts, CDs, mutual funds, stocks, and other liquid investments.

8. Review additional financial information documents to make a determination of the patient's liquid assets.

- Verify documents to make sure statements are not older than six months. If they are, request more recent statements from the patient.

- Sum the amounts in checking, saving accounts, CDs, mutual funds, stocks, and other liquid investments to obtain a liquid assets total.

Figure 7.7 | **Financial assistance determination procedure #10-20f (cont.)**

- If the liquid assets total amount is $10,000 or less, accounts(s) qualifies for financial assistance. Go to step nine.

- If the liquid assets total exceeds $10,000 and the excess over $10,000 is *more* than the outstanding balance, the patient does not qualify for financial assistance. Refer to policy #10-20d Payment Plan Resolution.

- If the liquid assets total exceeds $10,000 and the excess over $10,000 is *less* than the outstanding balance, the patient will owe the excess amount and the balance will qualify for financial assistance.

  Example:

	$15,000 investments	Outstanding balance	$20,000
less	$10,000	Less excess	$ 5,000
	$ 5,000	Eligible for financial assistance	$15,000
		Patient owes	$ 5,000

- Prepare partial eligibility letter to patient explaining the amount that qualified for financial assistance and the amount still owed. Refer to policy #10-20d Payment Plan Resolution for the amount still owed and proceed to step nine for amount eligible for financial assistance.

9. Attach the recommendation form along with account detail and forward accounts for approval. Approval levels for financial assistance write-offs are as follows:

- An account representative can initiate and approve any account balance up to $2,000. The collection supervisor will periodically review these accounts for accuracy.

- The collection supervisor will review and approve any account balance from $2,000 to $10,000 prior to write-off.

Figure **7.7**   **Financial assistance determination procedure
#10-20f (cont.)**

- The patient financial services manager will review and approve any account balance from $10,000 to $20,000 prior to write-off.

- The director of patient financial services will review and approve any account balance from $20,000 to $50,000 prior to write-off.

- The CFO will review and approve any account balance greater than $50,000 prior to write-off.

10. When approval is received, mail the patient a financial assistance approval letter or the previously prepared partial eligibility letter, whichever is applicable. Place a note on the patient's account in patient accounting system as to the level of financial assistance for which the patient is eligible.

11. Submit recommendation form to collection supervisor to write off to financial assistance adjustment code A9075.

Figure 7.8 **Discounted financial assistance for the uninsured #10-20g**

Department: Pre-registration services and patient financial services (PFS)

Policy: Uninsured patients expressing an inability to pay for medically necessary services at Hospital may be eligible to receive a discount. They must have previously met the qualifications established in the Financial Assistance Determination Policy #10-20f and have been determined ineligible based on income.

Purpose: To provide a consistent process for evaluating uninsured patients for the Hospital discounted financial assistance program.

Procedure:

1. After determining that the uninsured patient is ineligible for financial assistance according to policy #10-20f, use the adjusted annual income and compare the number of persons supported by total monthly income with the Expanded Income Level Guidelines.

   - If the adjusted annual income is equal to or below 200%, then the patient is eligible for a 50% discount. Proceed to step two.

   - If the adjusted annual income is above 200%, but is equal to or below 250%, then the patient is eligible for a 30% discount. Proceed to step two.

   - If the adjusted annual income falls above 250%, but is equal to or below 300%, then the patient is eligible for a 20% discount. Proceed to step two.

   - If the adjusted annual income is greater than 300%, then the patient does not qualify for discounted financial assistance. Refer to policy #10-20d Payment Plan Resolution.

2. Prepare a discounted financial assistance letter to the patient explaining the amount that qualified for discounted financial assistance and the amount still owed. Refer to policy #10-20d Payment Plan Resolution for the amount still owed and proceed to step three for the amount eligible for discounted financial assistance.

Figure 7.8 — Discounted financial assistance for the uninsured #10-20g (cont.)

3. Attach the recommendation form along with account detail and forward account for approval. Approval levels for discounted financial assistance write-offs are as follows:

- An account representative can initiate and approve any discount up to $2,000. The collection supervisor will periodically review these accounts for accuracy.

- The collection supervisor will review and approve any discount from $2,000 to $10,000 prior to write-off.

- The PFS manager will review and approve any discount from $10,000 to $20,000 prior to write-off.

- The director of PFS will review and approve any account balance from $20,000 to $50,000 prior to write-off.

- The CFO will review and approve any discount greater than $50,000 prior to write-off.

4. When approval is received, mail the patient the prepared discounted financial assistance letter. Place note on patient's account in the patient accounting system as to the level of discounted financial assistance for which the patient was eligible.

5. Submit recommendation form to collection supervisor to write off to partial financial assistance adjustment code A9076.

Figure 7.8	Discounted financial assistance for the uninsured #10-20g (cont.)

The revised income guidelines are as follows:

# Supported	150% level	200% level	250% level	300% level
1	$14,355	$19,140	$23,925	$28,710
2	$19,245	$25,660	$32,075	$38,490
3	$24,135	$32,180	$40,225	$48,270
4	$29,025	$38,700	$48,375	$58,050
5	$33,915	$45,220	$56,525	$67,830
6	$38,805	$51,740	$64,675	$77,610
7	$43,695	$58,260	$72,825	$87,390
8	$48,585	$64,780	$80,975	$97,170
For each additional person add:	$4,890	$6,520	$8,150	$9,780
Discount to be applied to charges	100%	50%	30%	20%

Impact of changes

Hospital implemented the revised charity and discounting policy on February 1, 2005. The anticipated impacts are an increase in charity write-offs and a decrease in bad debts, as well as an increase in patient satisfaction with Hospital's financial processes.

Case study 3: West Virginia University Hospitals and University Health Associates

Provider Internet profile

WVUH consists of Ruby Memorial Hospital, WVU Children's Hospital, Mary Babb Randolph Cancer Center, Jon Michael Moore Trauma Center, and Chestnut Ridge Hospital. University Health Associates (the teaching faculty practice) and specialized care facilities complete the profile.

Uncompensated care information

WVUH operates from revenues collected from patients, insurance companies, and other agencies. It receives no tax support. As a patient, you may request itemized billing and will receive monthly statements of your account with the hospital.

Our counselors and customer service staff are familiar with many programs that provide financial assistance and will help you apply for assistance. To be considered for any assistance, you will have to complete a financial statement.[4]

Charity-care issues

An opportunity existed between WVUH (acute care hospital) and UHA (physician practice) to redesign and implement an improved financial counseling process for patients. The charity process was an integral part of this opportunity. The hospital is an academic teaching facility with a closed medical practice plan adjacent to the facility. The acute care hospital and physician practice share the same patients. From 2002 to 2003, the self-pay collection opportunity had risen by more than 8% within the organizations. Industry trends indicated the growing dilemma of managing the self-pay patient population and that of the underinsured. The facilities could give patients one contact for financial counseling at both organizations. The facilities gained support from both senior managements to implement a joint charity-care program for the patient population. The facilities also retained an outside consulting firm to assist in the process improvement. There also existed the opportunity to appropriately shift bad debt accounts to charity and bad debt/charity to funded programs, thus improving the collection process for both organizations.

The organizations identified the following areas as barriers to efficiently and accurately processing patients' charity care applications:

Figure 7.9	WVUH and UHA statistical profile

WVUH profile	
Annual net revenue	$377,614,000
Provider type	University/teaching hospital
Bed size	522
Governance	Health system
Bad debt as % of net revenue (FY04)	5.0%
Charity as % of net revenue (FY04)	5.8%
UHA Profile	
Annual net revenue	$127,204,000
Provider type	Physician
Annual patient visits	417,000
Governance	Health system
Bad Debt as % of net revenue (FY04)	7.71%
Charity as % of net revenue (FY04)	3.75%

- Staffing
- Inconsistent guidelines between organizations
- Total manual paper process
- Inconsistent application of policy guidelines
- Lengthy appeal process for patients
- Inadequate reporting of workload volume, pending applications, denials
- No central repository of available funding programs

Staffing was not adequate to provide financial counseling and charity-care processing to the volumes of patients. There were also services identified, such as family medicine and psychiatry, that received no financial counseling. The staffing model consisted of the following for both the hospital and the physician group:

- One inpatient financial counselor for 438 staffed beds
- Three outpatient financial counselors for over 400,000 outpatient visits

As part of the redesign to assess the staffing barrier, the hospital completed a time study to identify the average time a financial counselor spent with a patient for inpatient and outpatient services, including both scheduled and unscheduled services. On average it required approximately 27 minutes for inpatient services and 10 minutes for outpatient services. The consultants compared this with their data and agreed that this was fairly industry consistent. Using the current payer mix by patient volumes, the facilities determined the number of patients that should receive financial counseling and potential charity-care processing. The following proposed staffing plan included all services and was approved by both organizations:

- Four inpatient financial counselors
- Six outpatient financial counselors

Inconsistent policy guidelines existed between the hospital and the physician practice. This inconsistency made it difficult for a financial counselor to communicate with the patient. Patients did not understand why they could qualify for different charity-care percentages from each organization (each organization had a different sliding scale). An analysis was performed on the partial charity-care write-offs for both organizations, and projections were made that illustrated the impact of eliminating the partial scale and simply going to 200% of the poverty guidelines for a total adjustment. Based on the assessment, both boards approved the elimination of the sliding scale and implementation of the 200% adjustment criteria.

The total manual process for charity-care processing made it difficult to track where a patient's charity application was in the charity process. If a patient called in to either the hospital or physician practice billing office, staff from one side did not have access to the financial application completed for the other. Once either the hospital or physician group approved an application, that approval was manually communicated to the other provider, and the appropriate charity adjustment recorded on the account. This manual process also led to inconsistency and subjectivity of staff reviewing the application. An internal audit validated the concerns with the manual process. This manual process also led to an inefficient appeal process. Because the organizations are spread across a large campus and across town, there were mail delays between staff involved in reviewing the applications. Management also found it difficult to monitor workload volumes, pending applications, and denials. Each financial counselor or collector had individual paper files with no centralization.

Charity-care processing changes

The facilities formed a project team that represented both organizations to design and implement a solution. By working with information technology, the team developed an online charity application. The team shared its proposed framework with both organizations' staffs for input before final development. The team built all charity policy rules in the application itself. Once testing was complete, the team developed a training module for all staff. The benefits of this new tool include the following:

- Eliminates the manual process

- Removes subjectivity during screening process

- Makes patient data/application available to all financial counselors, front desk staff, customer service representatives, collectors, and management

- Includes an auto-tracking process (date/time stamp)

- Assesses patient financials against criteria of more than 30 funding entities at local, state, and federal levels—patients required to apply for appropriate government program if referred by counselor

- Makes access to care limited to truly medically necessary services during screening process (e.g., services such as plastic surgery are excluded)—emergent care provided regardless of financial status

- Automatically notifies management staff electronically during appeal process

The following quote from one of the financial counselors best illustrates the improved tool:

With the implementation of the online charity care application has come many benefits. There is less confusion as to how the application is to be processed. The computer now calculates the income for us. Also, anyone with access can verify the status of an application by looking online. We also can easily help each other with pending applications—all we need to do is pull up the application online where the other financial counselor stopped.

The online system is one of the unique features of this charity process redesign effort. The following screen shots illustrate the comprehensive nature of the screening tool and the ease of use. Gaining the ability to store information in a repository central to both providers was a critical success factor.

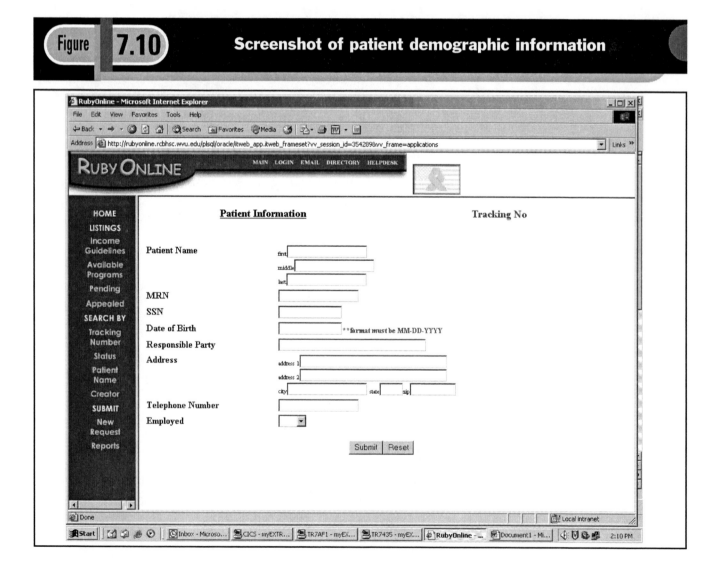

Figure 7.10 — Screenshot of patient demographic information

Figure 7.10 — Screenshot of household (family) information

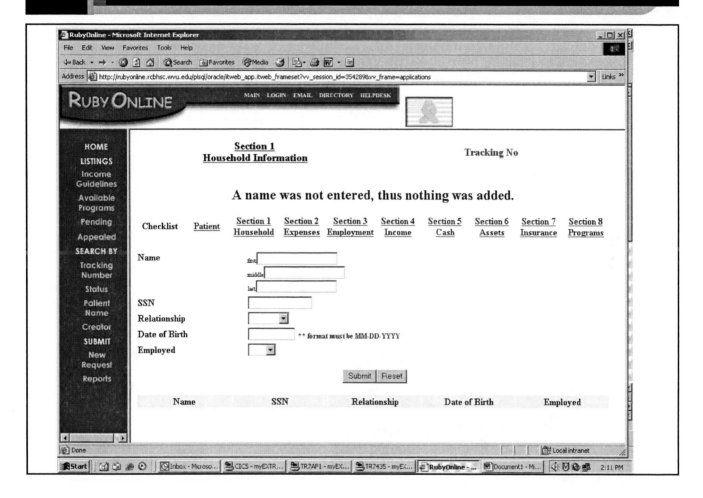

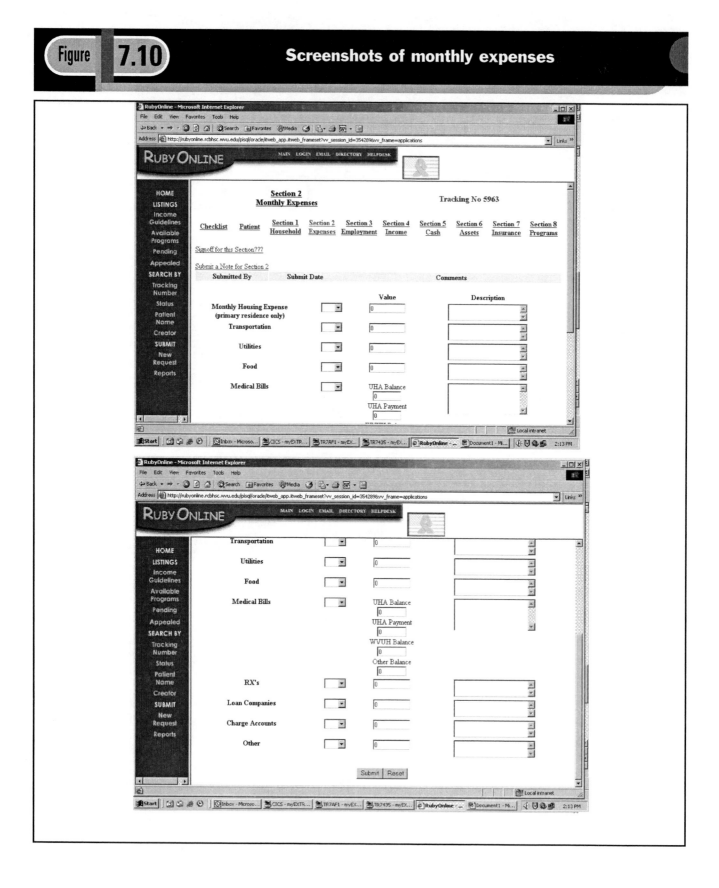

Figure 7.10 — Screenshots of monthly expenses

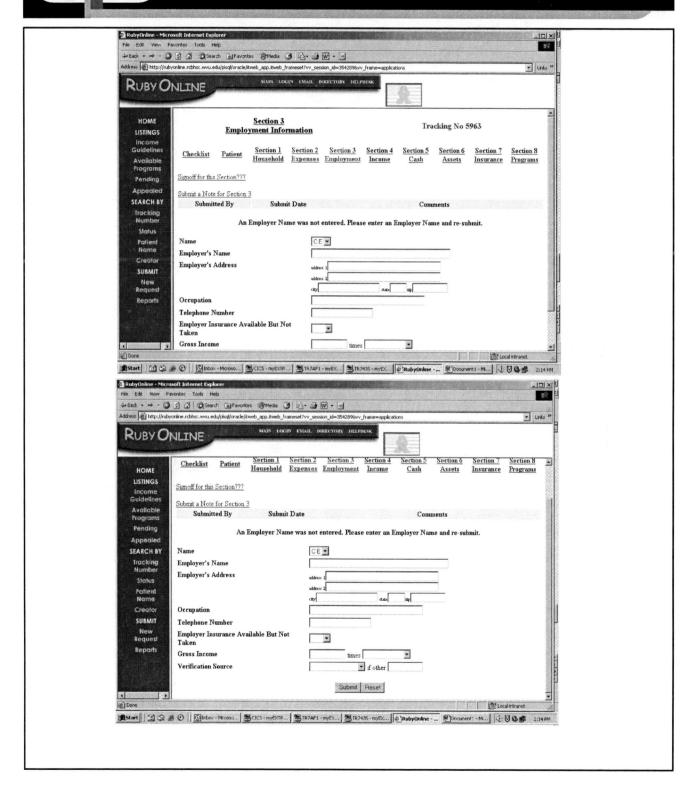

Figure 7.10 Screenshots of employment information

Figure 7.10 — Screenshot of other sources of income

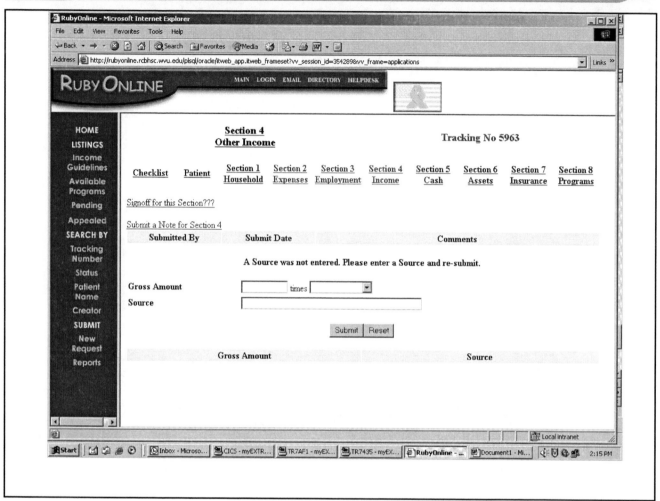

Figure	7.10	Screenshot of cash and related assets

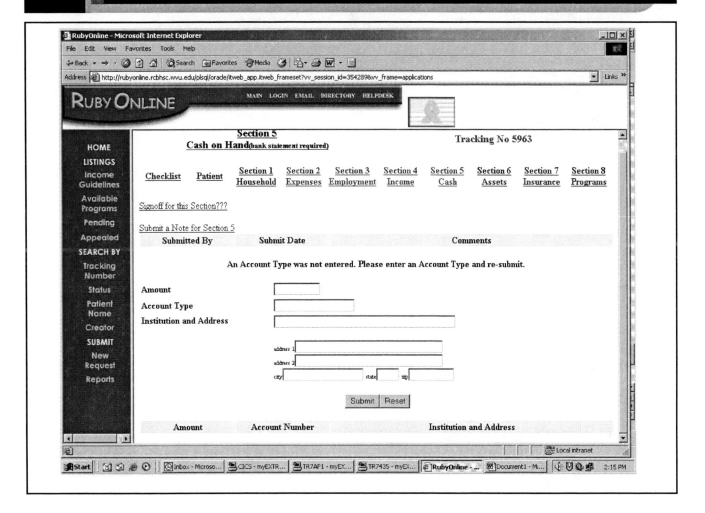

Figure 7.10   Screenshots of property and other assets

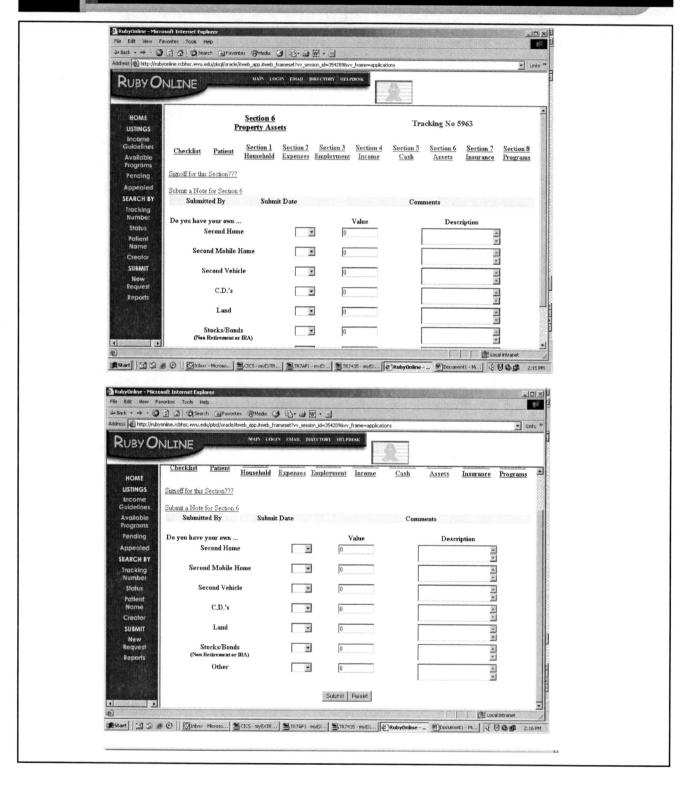

Figure 7.10 — Screenshot of insurance information

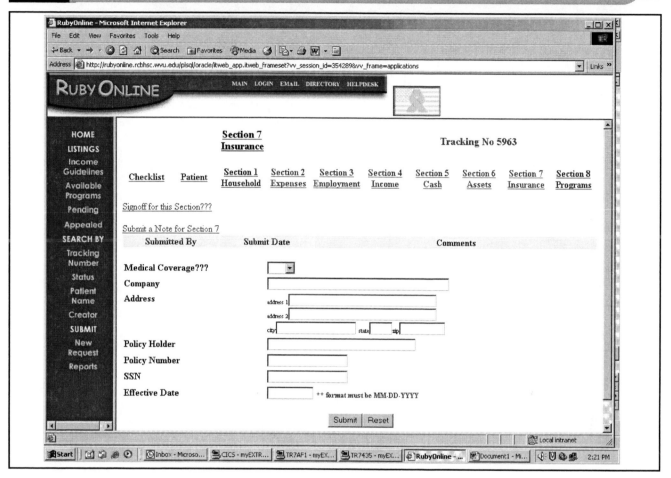

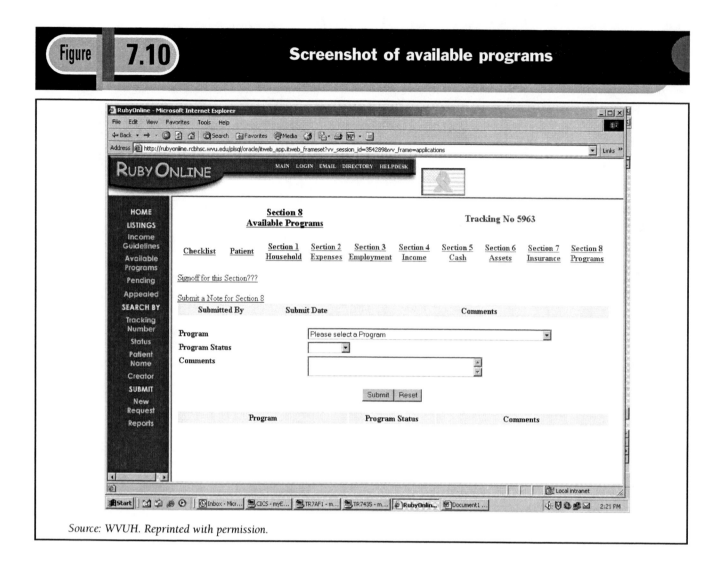

Figure 7.10 Screenshot of available programs

Source: WVUH. Reprinted with permission.

Impact of changes

Both organizations took a radical look and completed a major redesign in their approach to charity processing and financial counseling services. The organizations named the new program "Access WVU." The focus shifted to a pre-screening process with a goal to get patients qualified for alternate funding sources. Moving the screening and counseling process into the pre-service or time-of-service environment eliminated inefficient use of collector resources. Both organizations agreed to split the costs associated with the new program. For operational and reporting functions, the financial counselors would report the hospital patient access department.

To explain the program to patients, the organizations developed a financial counseling brochure for them. In addition, all financial counselors have business cards to give patients. With the ability to better manage and track the screening process, the physician practice developed a policy that repeat bad debtors who refuse to cooperate with financial counselors and the screening process may be dismissed from the practice. Although this may seem a small change in policy, it was a tremendous culture change.

The following statistics from the time period of January 2004–July 2004 illustrate part of the success of Access WVU:

- 2,995 patients screened
- 947 patients qualified for charity program
- 530 patients qualified for alternate source of funding

The upward trend of patient collection opportunity improved after implementation of the program. The program helps to identify other potential funding sources as well as patients eligible for charity. This graph shows the trend lines for both bad debt and charity. As expected, there has been a decrease in the bad debt percentage of net revenue, and the charity percentage of net revenue has increased. This confirms that the prior processes were not effective in correctly identifying charity v. bad debt accounts.

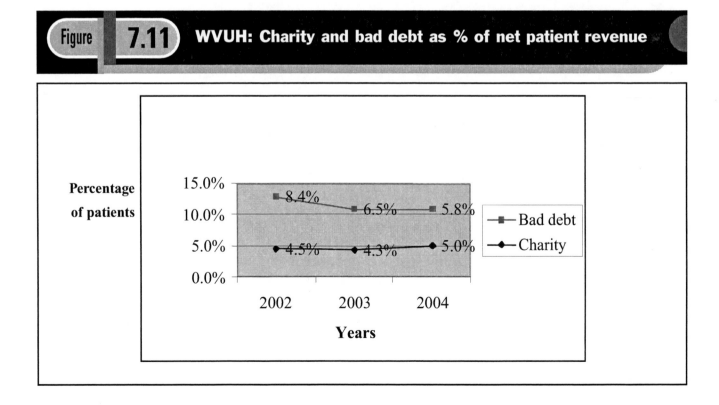

Figure 7.11 WVUH: Charity and bad debt as % of net patient revenue

Patient satisfaction was also a measurement of success. With the increase in financial counseling resources, the organization ranked best in practice with the patient satisfaction survey. The survey asked patients to rate satisfaction with the following statement in 2004: "The patient access staff clearly answered all your insurance and billing concerns." The organization scored a 95%, compared to a national norm of 82%, and best in class for the survey at 88%.

The restructuring of the charity program enabled both providers to manage the patient population more effectively with growing pressures of increased self-pay, increased copays/deductibles, and shrinking funding sources. The program has attained its goals and eliminated the barriers identified in the old charity processes.

Summary

These case studies illustrate changes in poverty guidelines and processing requirements, the application of technology, the movement of processing activity from the post-service process to the pre-service process, and the value of coordinated efforts to standardize charity processing within related organizations. For contact information about any of the case study participants, contact the author via e-mail at *swolfskill@cs.com*.

Notes

1. *www.ccmh.com.*

2. Revenue Cycle Partners in Billings, MT, Working Document, 2005.

3. Hospital's Web site. Anonymous.

4. *www.health.wvu.edu.*